THE ART OF MEDICINE

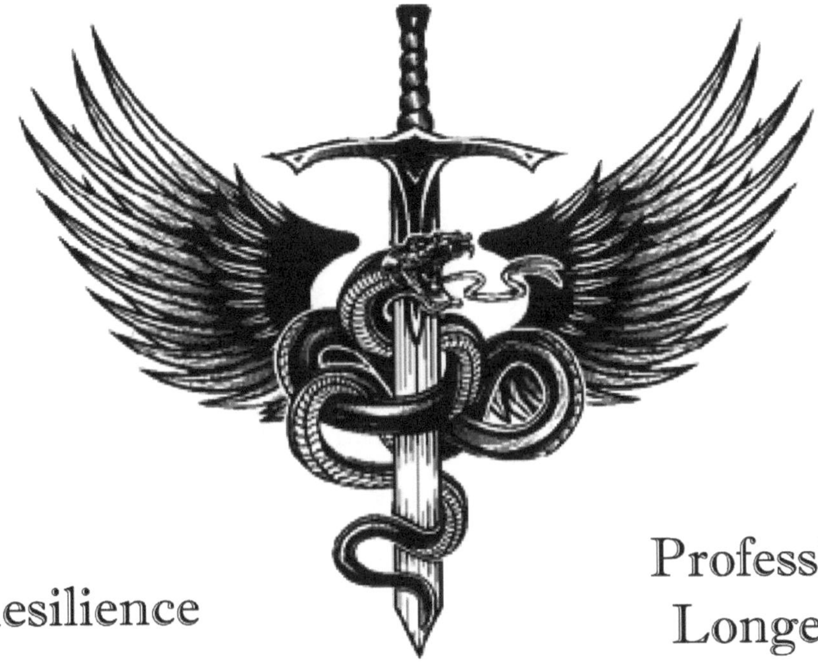

Resilience   Professional Longevity

A Warriors Mindset

A WARRIORS PROFESSION

Developing A Warriors Mindset
to Cultivate Resilience and Professional Longevity

Johnnie L. Gilpen Jr MHS MS PA-C CAQ(EM) NRP

Leslie J. Ballenger DrPH

Developing a Warrior's Mindset to Cultivate Resilience and Professional Longevity

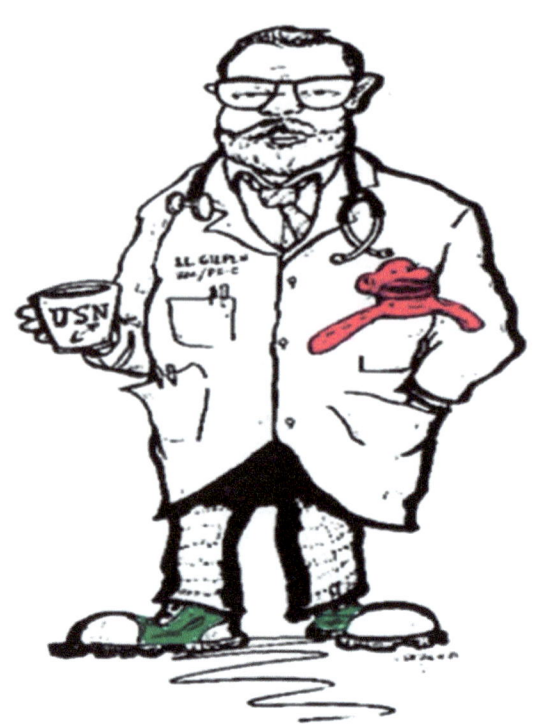

Copyright © 2025 Johnnie L. Gilpen Jr

Cartoons provided by Robert "Bob" Creager Copyright © 2025 Robert Creager

Graphics by Huma Rafeeq (creative artist) dezinsolutions.net

All rights reserved. No portion of this book may be reproduced, stored in a retrieval system, or transmitted in any form or by any means – electronic, mechanical, photocopy, recording, scanning, or other – except for brief quotations in critical reviews or articles, without the prior written permission of the publisher and the author.

Published by 8404 Publishing, LLC (www.8404publishing.com),

    Three Strand Warriors, LLC (www.3strandwarriorshealth.com) & (www.johnniegilpen.com)

Library of Congress Cataloging-in-Publication Data

Gilpen, Johnnie L. Jr, 1971 –

Ballenger, Leslie J. 1968 –

    The Art of Medicine – A Warriors Profession: Developing A Warriors Mindset for Cultivating Resilience and Professional Longevity Workbook / Johnnie L. Gilpen Jr. & Leslie J. Ballenger

Includes bibliographical references.

ISBN: 979-8-9918162-0-5

The Art of Medicine – A Warriors Profession™

TABLE OF CONTENTS

Table of Contents 3
   Special Thanks to the Pat Tillman Foundation..6
      Becoming a Tillman Scholar: Honoring a Legacy of Service and Leadership................6
Authors Note:..7
4-Hour Course Description...9
   Course Description: 9
   Target Audience:..9
   Scope of Course: 10
   Educational Credits: 10
No Barriers Life 11
   Core Beliefs: The 7 Life Elements 11
   Implementation of Life Elements 12
Summits 13
   Evolution One: Identifying Your Life Summits 13
      Evolution One Objectives: 14
      Evolution One Exercises: 17
         Exercise 1. A: 17
            Worksheet 1. A: Identifying Your Life Summits 18
         Exercise 1. B: 19
        Worksheet 1. B: Resilience Data Point #1 20
            Worksheet 1. B: Resilience Data Point #2 21

Developing a Warrior's Mindset to Cultivate Resilience and Professional Longevity

- Worksheet 1. B: Resilience Data Point #3 22
- Exercise 1. C: 23
- Exercise 1. D: 23

Rope Team 25

Evolution Two: Who's in My Foxhole? 25

- Evolution Two Objectives: 26
- Evolution Two: Exercises: 27
  - Exercise 2. A: 27
    - Worksheet 2. A: Identifying my Current Fighting Position 28
  - Exercise 2. B: 29
    - Worksheet 2. B: Describing My Current Fighting Position 30
    - Worksheet 2. B: Describing My Current Fighting Position 31
  - Exercise 2. C: 32
    - Worksheet 2. C: Identifying My Foxhole Buddies 33
  - Exercise 2. D: 34
    - Worksheet 2. D: Characteristics of My Foxhole Buddy # 1 34
    - Worksheet 2. D: Characteristics of My Foxhole Buddy # 2 35
  - Exercise 2. E: 35
  - Exercise 2. F: 36

Vision 37

Evolution Three: Defining Your Vision 37

- Evolution Three Objectives: 38
- Evolution Three Exercises: 39
  - Exercise 3. A: 39

Exercise 3. B: 43

    Worksheet 3. B: Building my Vision Cairn 44

Exercise 3. C: 45

Exercise 3. D: 46

References 48

    Publisher Contact Information 49

Appendix 51

Appendix A: Book List 52

Appendix B: OK First Responder Wellness Division 53

Appendix C: Worksheets 55

    Worksheet 1. A: Identifying Your Life's Summits 56

    Worksheet 1. B: Resilience Data Point #1 57

    Worksheet 1. B: Resilience Data Point #2 58

    Worksheet 1. B: Resilience Data Point #3 59

    Worksheet 2. A: Identifying My Current Fighting Position 60

    Worksheet 2. B: Describing My Current Fighting Position 61

    Worksheet 2. B: Describing My Current Fighting Position 62

    Worksheet 2. C: Identifying Who's In My Foxhole 63

    Worksheet 2. D: Characteristics of My Foxhole Buddy # 1 64

    Worksheet 2. D: Characteristics of My Foxhole Buddy # 2 65

    Exercise 3. A: Prompt Box 66

    Worksheet 3. A: My Values Brain Mapping Box 67

    Worksheet 3. B: Building My Vision Cairn 68

Special Thanks to the Pat Tillman Foundation

Becoming a Tillman Scholar: Honoring a Legacy of Service and Leadership

As a Tillman Scholar, I'm part of a community inspired by Pat Tillman's selfless act of serving in the US Army after 9/11. Pat, a former NFL safety who played for the Arizona Cardinals from 1998 to 2001, put his football career on hold to serve his country. The Pat Tillman Foundation empowers remarkable leaders, active-duty service members, veterans, and military spouses who drive impact worldwide.

The Foundation was founded in 2004 by Pat's friends and family. Since then, it has built a network of nearly 1,000 Tillman Scholars. The Foundation cultivates a lifelong network of leaders who share Pat Tillman's values of scholarship, humble leadership, service, and impact. I'm proud to be among the Tillman Scholars community, dedicated to positively impacting the world.

To learn more about the Pat Tillman Foundation and the Tillman Scholar Program and how you can get involved, please visit www.PatTillmanFoundation.org.

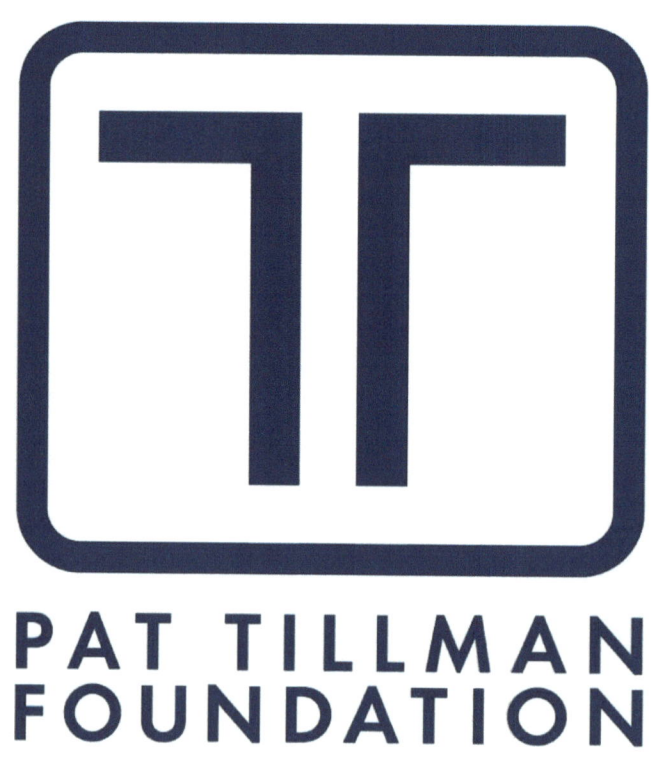

AUTHORS NOTE:

There is no such thing as a new idea. It is impossible. We simply take a lot of old ideas and put them into a sort of mental kaleidoscope. We give them a turn and they make new and curious combinations. We keep on turning and making new combinations indefinitely, but they are the same old pieces of colored glass that have been in use through all the ages."(Paine, 2018)   *- Mark Twain*

This workbook is adapted from the **No Barriers Warriors Program**, which I was fortunate to participate in during the COVID-19 Pandemic. It helped keep me grounded as I slogged through the craziness of the Emergency Room. This is only possible through the gracious kindness of my friend and co-founder of No Barriers, Erik Weihenmayer, who permitted me to bend the material to healthcare workers and First Responders, including Emergency Medical Services (EMS), Fire, Law Enforcement, and 911 Dispatch. As such, we are introducing a new group of people to the concept and belief that **What's Within You Is Stronger Than What's in Your Way**. Thank you, Erik!

I also want to thank my friend, mentor, brother in this life, fellow emergency medicine PA, and co-founder of No Barriers, Jeff Evans, for encouraging and motivating me and believing in yet another crazy idea – I appreciate you!

To my wife, there is never enough gratitude and appreciation for your work. If it were not for you—you are my rock, my foundation, my strength to draw from, my clarity when I have none, and the finesse to everything I do—none of this would ever have come to fruition.

Thank you to all the men and women I have served with over my 30 years of public service - it is an honor.

My brother, Rob Creager, from a different mother, has graciously provided the doodles for this program. I have been blessed with amazing people in my life, and for almost 30 years, Rob has supported, dragged, carried, encouraged, and laughed with me and often at me, picked me up when I have fallen, and followed me on more crazy adventures than I can remember. Thanks for always being there, brother!

To Dr. Kendall Luyt, M.D., and Dr. Ryan Butchee, M.D., February and March 2023 will be two months I will never forget. Those patients are etched in my heart, along with many others, but those kids are branded such that they are eternal next to my Marines, Corpsman, and Soldiers. I am grateful that I had the honor of not just working; it was more than just working, it was serving alongside both of you. You two were a major catalyst for what this has become. I am genuinely thankful for the mentoring you both have provided and for the grace and kindness you have shown me. I am also grateful for all the First Responders I have served with and alongside over my thirty-year career. Thank you all!

Lastly, thank you to my mentors, to those who continue to support my *crazy ideas*, to those mentors I have never met, and to those I have yet to meet… the list is long – Terry Weaver, Harry Whitlock, Ryan Brown, Curtis Knoles, Brad Lancaster, my uncles - Alive, Jr., Rick, Ed, and Bennie, David Epstein, David Goggins, Jocko Willink, Joe De Sena, Andy Frisella, Dwayne Johnson, Tony Robbins, Tim Ferris, Joesph Campbell, Napoleon Hill, Tom Lillig and David Shurna, Steve Pressfield, Sun Tzu, Ernest Hemingway, Theodore Roosevelt, John C. Maxwell, Pat Tillman, and EVERY SINGLE TILLMAN SCHOLAR.

Thrive, Don't Just Survive!

JG

Johnnie L Gilpen Jr PA-C CAQ (EM) NRP

Union City, Oklahoma

23rd August 2024

The Art of Medicine – A Warriors Profession™

4-Hour Course Description

Course Description:

This 4-hour course aims to teach Healthcare Professionals – including, but not limited to, physicians, physician assistants, nurse practitioners, behavioral health providers, allied health professionals, volunteers, and First Responders – to utilize Life Element-based resilience tools and skills. These tools are crucial for managing personal and professional stress, burnout, and empathy fatigue. They are designed with a strong focus on promoting self-care strategies. Burnout often manifests as emotional exhaustion, depersonalization, and a diminished sense of personal accomplishment, resulting in a significant decline in job satisfaction and effectiveness. Compassion fatigue and chronic stress contribute to this burnout, ultimately affecting practitioners' well-being and patient care. By prioritizing self-care and stress management, you can mitigate these effects, improve personal and professional fulfillment, and enhance overall health and patient outcomes. By strengthening these skills, you can reduce practitioner stress, professional impairment, and occupational burnout, and positively impact patient outcomes, as well as your health and life outside of work.

Target Audience:

By enrolling in this program, Healthcare Professionals and First Responders will gain valuable skills and knowledge in managing personal and professional stress, burnout, and empathy fatigue. This course is designed to enhance their ability to thrive in their professional and personal lives.

Scope of Course:

The Art of Medicine – A Warrior's Profession Course:
- This 4-hour course is designed for the requesting organization.
- Addresses the unique healthcare on-the-job dangers (i.e., highly infectious diseases, active shooters, mass casualties), shift creep, professional burnout/stress, and suicide among healthcare and first responders.
- Assist participants in developing resources and support tools that help build resiliency and perseverance and promote professional longevity.

Educational Credits:

Public Health Research and Education Associates LLC (PHREA) awards 4.0 Continuing Education Units (CEU) (4-hour Course) for:
- ✓ Licensed Professional Counselors (LPC) and Licensed Marriage and Family Therapists (LMFT) by the Oklahoma Board of Behavioral Health Licensure,
- ✓ Licensed Social Workers (LSW) by the Oklahoma Board of Licensed Social Workers
- ✓ Licensed Alcohol and Drug Counselors (LADC) by the Oklahoma Board of Licensed Alcohol and Drug Counselors,
- ✓ CEUs for Paramedics and EMTs, and
- ✓ 2 hours Mental Health CEs for Law Enforcement approved by the Oklahoma Council on Law Enforcement Education and Training (CLEET).

Contact: For more information or to book a class, contact Dr. Leslie Ballenger at 405-633-1190 or info@johnnniegilpen or artofmedicine@3strandwarriors.com.

NO BARRIERS LIFE

What's within you is stronger than what's in your way... - *No Barriers Motto*

Core Beliefs: The 7 Life Elements

VISION — Define a purpose that inspires you to give your best back to the world.

PIONEER — Persevere through challenges to innovate.

ALCHEMY — Harness life experience into optimism.

REACH — Move beyond your comfort zone to grow and reach your goals.

ROPE TEAM — Collaborate and connect with others to build strong communities.

SUMMITS — Find the gifts earned through the struggle.

ELEVATE — Impact the world as a leader who serves.

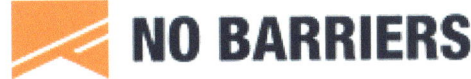

https://nobarriersusa.org/

Implementation of Life Elements

This four-hour course will examine the first three (3) life elements: **SUMMITs**, **ROPE TEAM**, and **VISION**. We have broken down **ROPE TEAM** into two (2) components: the first, which we cover in this course—FOXHOLE BUDDIES, and the second, developing both personal and professional **ROPE TEAMs**. We also offer **The Art of Medicine – Beyond Your Vision**, part two of the course, which covers the second half of ROPE TEAMs: **REACH**, **PIONEERING**, **ALCHEMY**, and **ELEVATE**.

For further information, please visit our website at http://www.johnniegilpen.com or contact Dr. Leslie Ballenger at (405) 633-1190 or via email at info@johnniegilpen.com. Johnnie Gilpen, PA-C CAQ(EM) NRP, can be reached at johnnie@johnniegilpen.com or (405) 919-9511.

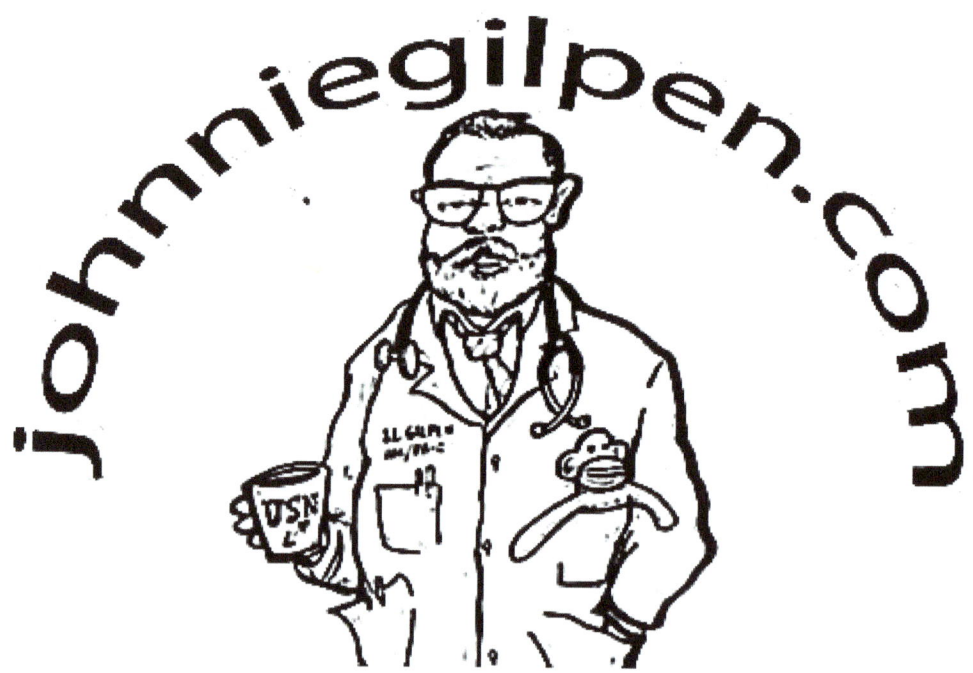

SUMMITS

> *"In my life I want to create passion in my own life and with those I care for. I want to feel, experience and live every emotion. I will suffer through the bad for the heights of the good."*
> — Pat Tillman

Evolution One: Identifying Your Life Summits

The life element, **SUMMITs**, aims to help you reflect on your life experiences to find the gifts you have earned through struggle. We refer to these gifts as Resilience Data Points, RDPs for short. They are the "Rocky" moments in your life – when Apollo Creed has you on the 'ropes'… then you are on the mat. In your head, you hear Mickey saying, "Down, down, stay down." Nevertheless, you find that inner strength to climb the ropes and 'go the distance.' We have all had those moments when others did not believe we could achieve our goals… moments when we did not think we would reach our goals. Our **SUMMITs** can be significant and victorious, such as completing the Bataan Death March Marathon. The October 2019 issue of Men's Health called it "The Toughest Race in America." The race motto is "More than just a marathon – No Mama, No Pappa, No Uncle Sam," a reference to statements made by the defenders of Bataan in the Philippines during the Japanese invasion in WWII. The race is a 26-mile ruck, military slang for a hike, through the New Mexico desert and mountains with a 2,600 ft total elevation climb, a 30 lb. rucksack or backpack, your food, water, and "other gear" as needed. With the help and motivation of eight (8) fellow Tillman Scholars, I finished in 13 hours and 3 minutes, well over their recommended 8-hour goal. However, my goal was not to win but to cross the finish line, whether walking, stumbling, or crawling, and not die, or climbing to 12,464 feet 63 days post spinal surgery. It was an endeavor in both resilience and perseverance. These moments are essential to our personal growth. We can draw strength from them when we are "on the ropes" in the future.

On the other hand, they can be small but significant moments in our lives. Did you reach a point you thought would be impossible? Run further than you ever have? Pass the neurology test you have dreaded, or maybe something nobody knows about but you? **SUMMITs** can identify those moments that are high points in our lives outside of our goals, just surprises along the trail to the **SUMMIT**. Celebrating your life story's big and small moments is vital to recognize where you came from and where you can grow. ("Summits - No Barriers Warriors," 2020).

In this evolution, the participants will be provided with simple tools to help them repurpose their **SUMMITS**, repackaging them into FUEL that can be used repeatedly to draw strength when needed.

Evolution One Objectives:

1. **REFLECT** on the participant's life, specifically, the high points– those 'Rocky' moments, which we refer to as **SUMMITs**. **IDENTIFY** three (3) to six (6) Summits (AKA – Resilience Data Points (RDP)).

2. **DESCRIBE** up to six (6) of the participants' most significant **SUMMITs** using a simple single sentence for each achievement.

3. For three (3) of the participants' most significant **SUMMITs** (to them) identified in OBJECTIVE 1.
   1. **Identify**
      a) the DATE when the **SUMMIT** occurred,
      b) WHERE the participant was when they reached each specific **SUMMIT**,
      c) WHO the participant was when they reached each of the **SUMMITS**,
      d) Summarily **DESCRIBE** WHY the participant was pursuing each of the **SUMMITs**,
      e) **DESCRIBE** and **DISCUSS** any significant OBSTACLES the participant had to overcome to reach each of the **SUMMITs** and

f) **IDENTIFY** those HATERS who did not believe the participant would complete their goal to use as FUEL for the future.

4. Using the three (3) Resilience Data Point (RDP) Cards provided, the participant will kick start their own personal Cookie Jar by **TRANSCRIBING** the information **IDENTIFIED** in OBJECTIVE 1.3 onto the RDP cards.

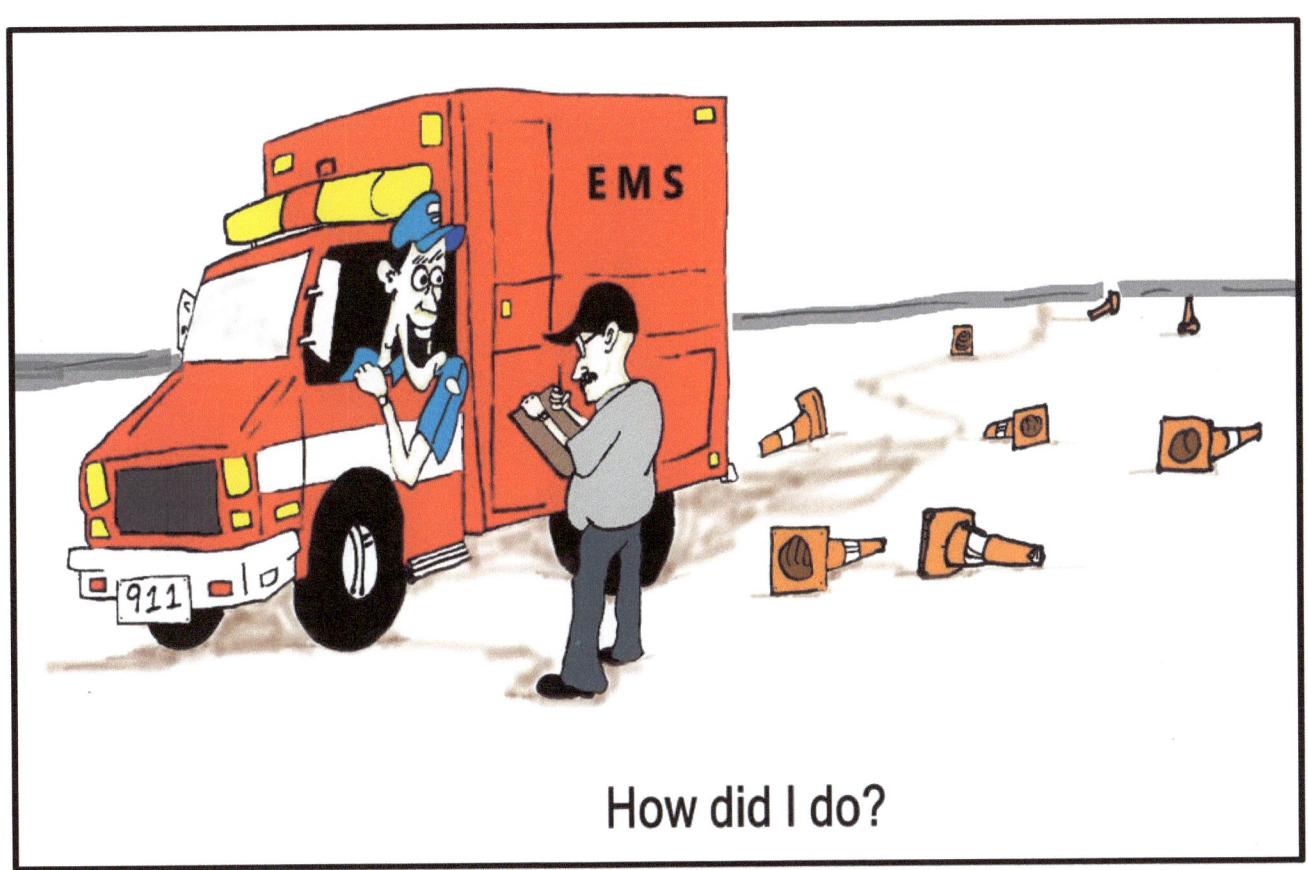

Developing a Warrior's Mindset to Cultivate Resilience and Professional Longevity

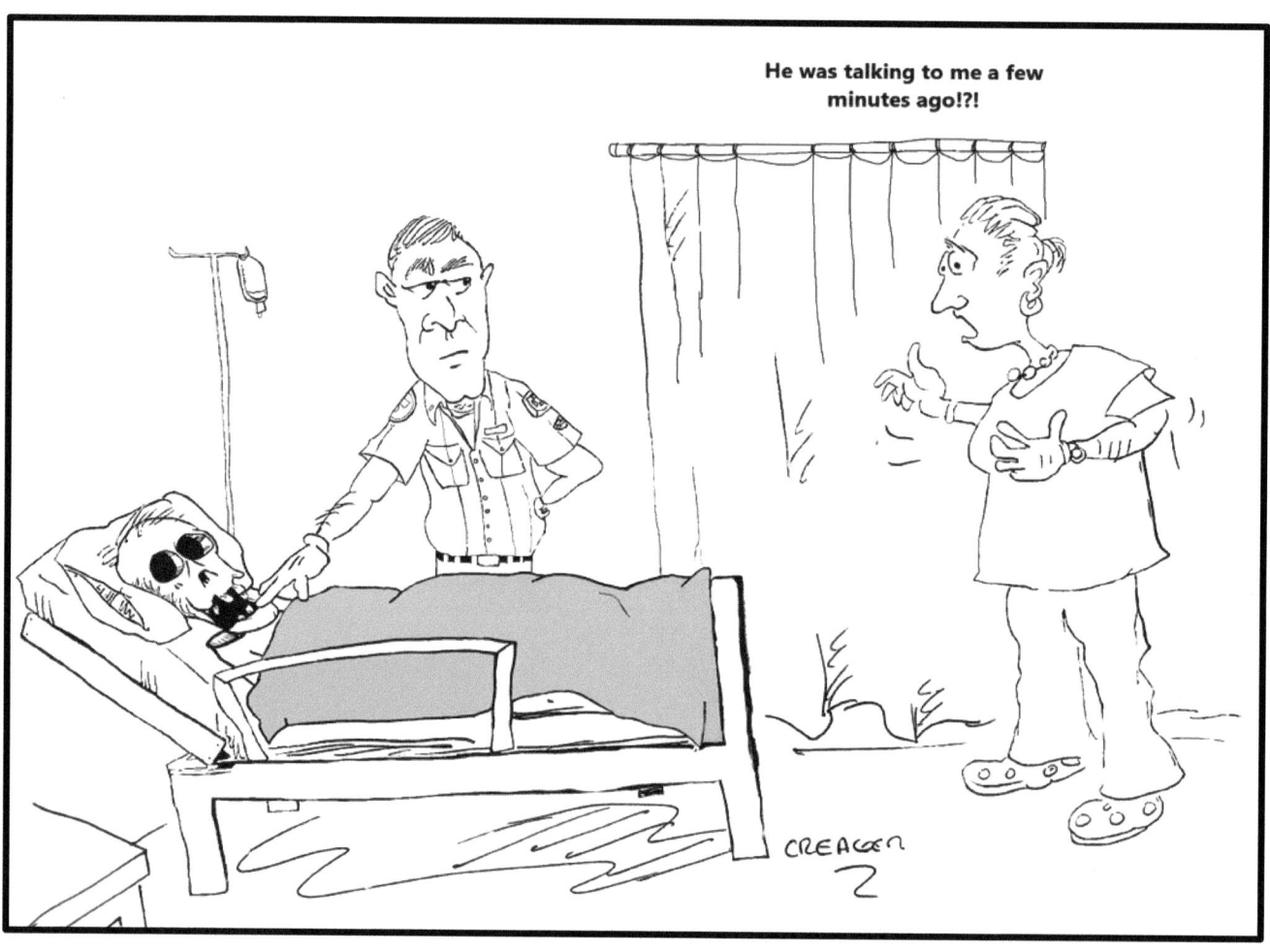

Perseverance

The Art of Medicine – A Warriors Profession™

SUMMITS

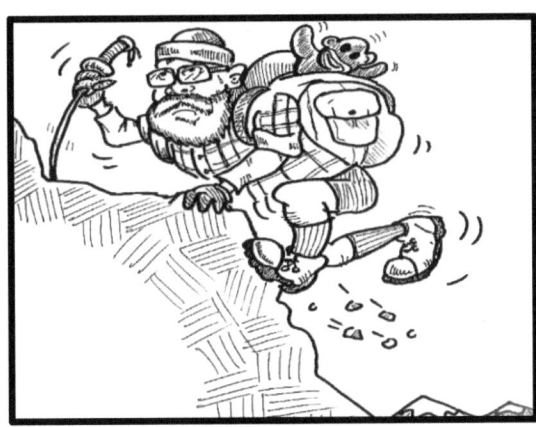

Evolution One: Identifying Your Life Summits

Evolution One Exercises:

Exercise 1. A: The purpose of the life element, **SUMMITs**, is to help you reflect on your life experiences to find the gifts you have earned through struggle. Our SUMMITS can be prominent and victorious, or they can also be small but high points in the middle of chasing our dreams. SUMMITS are our Resilience Data Points (RDP) – the points in life upon which we build our resilience (De Sena & Pence, 2021). Reflect on your life, specifically the high points – the **SUMMITs** and achievements, and identify at least three (3) but try to identify six (6) of your highest **SUMMITs**. Think of those that have the most meaning to you.

DESCRIBE these achievements in the blocks provided in Worksheet 1. A: Identifying Your Life Summits using a simple single sentence. (*Additional worksheets are provided in the appendix section.*) Just write; they do not have to be in any order or significance. They can be **SUMMITs** everyone knows about or something you have kept to yourself… do not worry about grammar, syntax, or spelling. Start writing.

WORKSHEET 1. A: IDENTIFYING YOUR LIFE SUMMITS

Identifying Your Life Summits — My Summits

1.

2.

3.

4.

5.

6.

Perseverance

Exercise 1. B: Using the three (3) Resilience Data Points #1-3 worksheets, **DESCRIBE** three (3) of your life's most significant **SUMMITs** you identified in EXERCISE 1. A. Using a few brief sentences, **DESCRIBE** –

a) WHEN reached each **SUMMIT** (the DATE: month, and year at minimum),

b) WHERE you were when the event happened,

   c) WHOM helped you reach each of the **SUMMITs**,

d) WHY you were pursuing these **SUMMITs**,

e) Any OBSTACLES that you had to overcome to reach each of the **SUMMITs** and

f) **LIST** your HATERS – those who did not believe in you. This can be a powerful motivational FUEL!

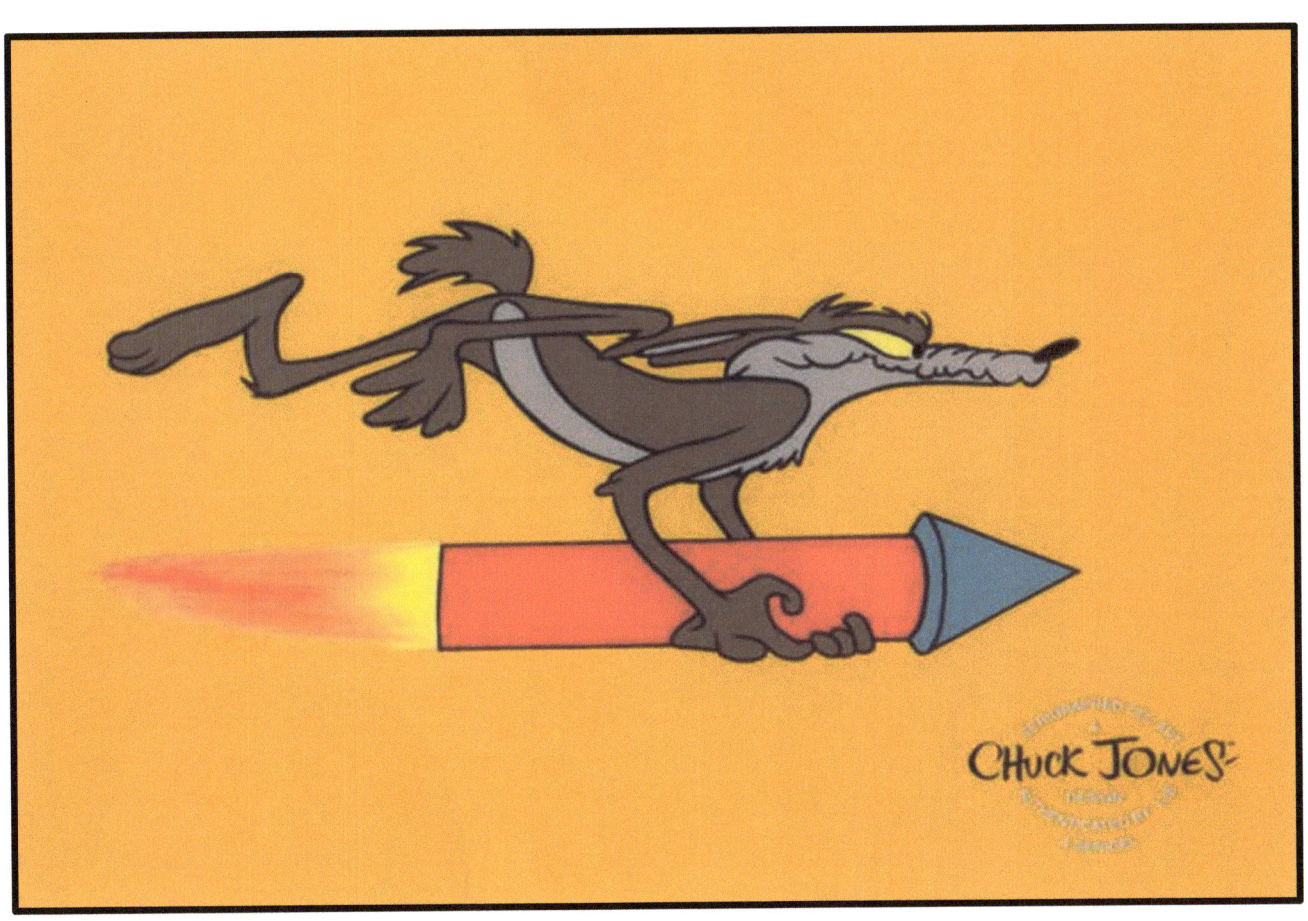

Worksheet 1. B: Resilience Data Point #1

| Resilience Data Point **#1** |

Your Summit #1

When?

Where Were You?

Who Were You With?

Why Was This Summit So Significant?

What Obstacles Did You Overcome?

Perseverance

WORKSHEET 1, B: RESILIENCE DATA POINT #2

Resilience Data Point #2

Your Summit #2

- When?
- Where Were You?
- Who Were You With?
- Why Was This Summit So Significant?

What Obstacles Did You Overcome?

Resilience

WORKSHEET 1, B: RESILIENCE DATA POINT #3

Resilience Data Point #3

Your Summit #3

When?

Where Were You?

Who Were You With?

Why Was This Summit So Significant?

What Obstacles Did You Overcome?

Exercise 1. C: Please **TRANSCRIBE** the information from the three (3) **SUMMITs** you identified in EXERCISE 1. B to the three (3) Resilience Data Point (RDP) Cards in the Cookie Jar provided. These will be the foundation to get your Cookie Jar started. It will be up to you to continue adding more **SUMMITs** to your Cookie Jar and fill it with your past performances. (Future Summits – AKA Resilience Data Points (De Sena & Pence, 2021))

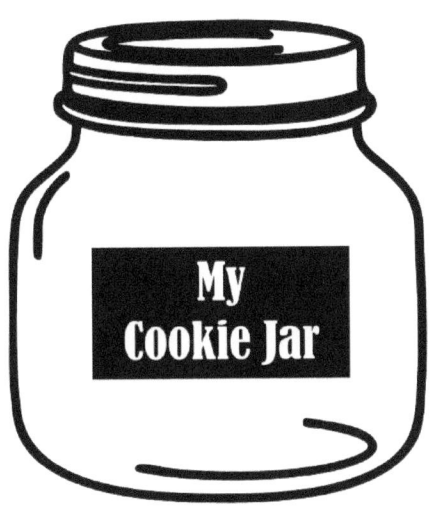

Exercise 1. D: A foundational pillar of positive psychology is the active practice of GRATITUDE. Practicing gratitude is genuinely appreciating all the people in our lives, such as our family, friends, neighbors, and co-workers; our health, our jobs and careers, and our achievements – the list is endless and different for everyone. Take a few moments and **REFLECT** on the people in your life who were there to help you reach the **SUMMITs DESCRIBED** in EXERCISE 1. B. Take the next few minutes to either **TEXT** these people and **THANK** them for their support and help – and/or **MAKE** a social media post on your favorite platform (Facebook, X, Instagram, etc.) thanking the people who have helped you reach your goals. Never underestimate your impact on those individuals who have helped you, their family and friends, those around you, and those you do not know. You never know who is watching you. Let others see the act of gratitude; help others see the success and power of your life's **SUMMITs**. Use the following hashtags: **gratitudeARTMED   #ARTMEDWarriorProf   #SummitsARTMED   #NobarriersARTMED   #PTF-ARTMED**

Developing a Warrior's Mindset to Cultivate Resilience and Professional Longevity

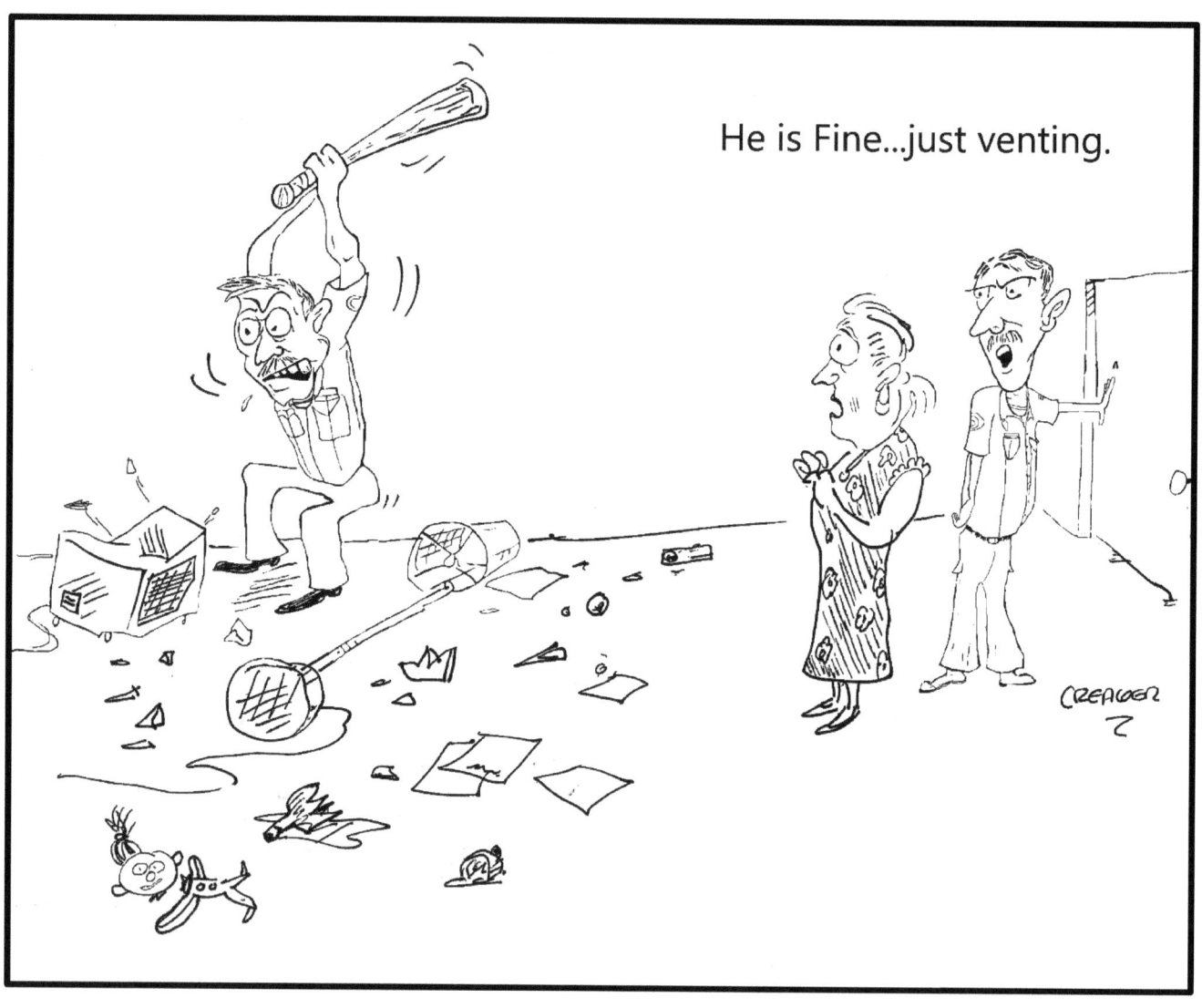

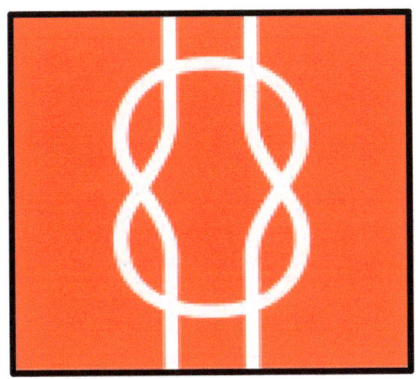

ROPE TEAM

"Two people are better off than one, for they can help each other succeed. If one person falls, the other can reach out and help. But someone who falls alone is in real trouble." — Ecclesiastes 4:9-10(NLT)

Evolution Two: Who's in My Foxhole?

The life element, **ROPE TEAM**, aims to help you identify the people around you WHO will help you accomplish your goal(s). This group is not just a general list of your friends and close family members. It is a specially curated list of individuals with specific gifts, talents, and drive to help you when your goal seems too far off or challenging. This is a team to collaborate with – the people who know you, those who will call you back to your vision when you start to veer away from it, and just as important, individuals who will be there celebrating with you all the way to the end. They do not have to be family, colleagues, or lifelong friends. These people do not have to be all the same, but should be uniquely different. ("Rope Team - No Barriers Warriors," 2020).

Developing a Warrior's Mindset to Cultivate Resilience and Professional Longevity

Evolution Two Objectives:

1. **CONDUCT** an inner reflection and **IDENTIFY** the type of personal mental fighting position the participant most often finds themselves fighting from – a One-MAN FIGHTING POSITION, a Two-MAN FOXHOLE, or a Three-MAN FOXHOLE?

2. (A) For the participant who commonly finds themselves fighting from a One-MAN FIGHTING POSITION, **DEFINE** and **DESCRIBE** the pros and cons of their situation. Also, **IDENTIFY** and **EXPLAIN** why the participant is predominantly in a ONE-MAN FIGHTING POSITION.

   or

   (B) If the participant(s) *seldom* find themselves in a One-MAN FIGHTING POSITION, **IDENTIFY** a situation where the participant fought alone in a One-MAN FIGHTING POSITION, then **DESCRIBE** how they faired through that specific situation.

3. **IDENTIFY** two (2) individuals the participant wants in their foxhole to fight with who the participant is willing to reciprocate. **DEFINE** and **DESCRIBE** the characteristics of why the participant has chosen these two individuals.

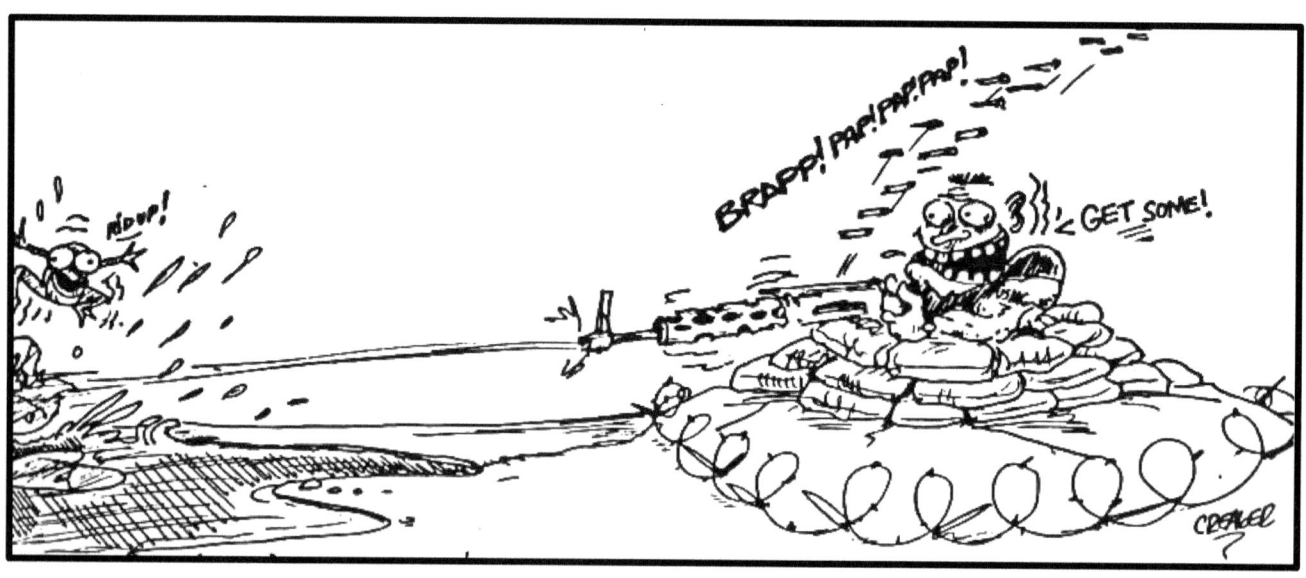

Perseverance

ROPE TEAM

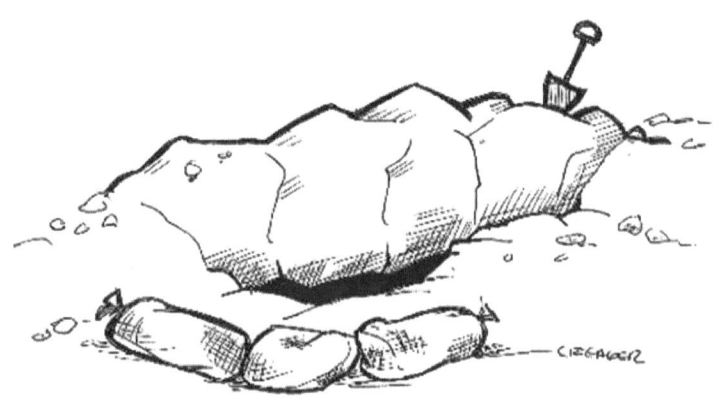

Evolution Two: My Fighting Position – Who's in My Foxhole & Why?

Evolution Two: Exercises:

Exercise 2. A: In life, we all develop some form of a mental foxhole – a fighting position from which to take on the world around us. For those who have never had the 'pleasure' of digging a foxhole, they are physically small, cramped, uncomfortable spaces meant to hold up to three people at the most. Unfortunately, many people turn their foxholes into One-MAN FIGHTING POSITIONS. The One-Man FIGHTING POSITION is meant to be temporary. It is not intended to be long-term – dig in, stay, and play, hang your hat kind of places. Becoming isolated in these one-man fighting death traps does not take long. They are lonely places. If we are not careful, they become our graves (Goggins, 2022).

Let us take a moment to **SELF-REFLECT**, look inward, as David Goggins says, do a "live autopsy" on ourselves, and think about our current mental fighting position. Dig deep, look into your 'accountability mirror" – which fighting position do you spend most of your time fighting in... a Three-MAN FOXHOLE or a One-MAN FIGHTING POSITION? (Goggins, 2018)

On <u>Worksheet 2. A: Identifying my Current Fighting Position</u>, please **WRITE** today's date at the top of the circle of the fighting position you currently find yourself in. Some of you may have never thought about it in this context. You may not have a fighting position, which is also okay. This is just a tool to help you **IDENTIFY** a reference starting point from which you can work.

WORKSHEET 2. A: IDENTIFYING MY CURRENT FIGHTING POSITION

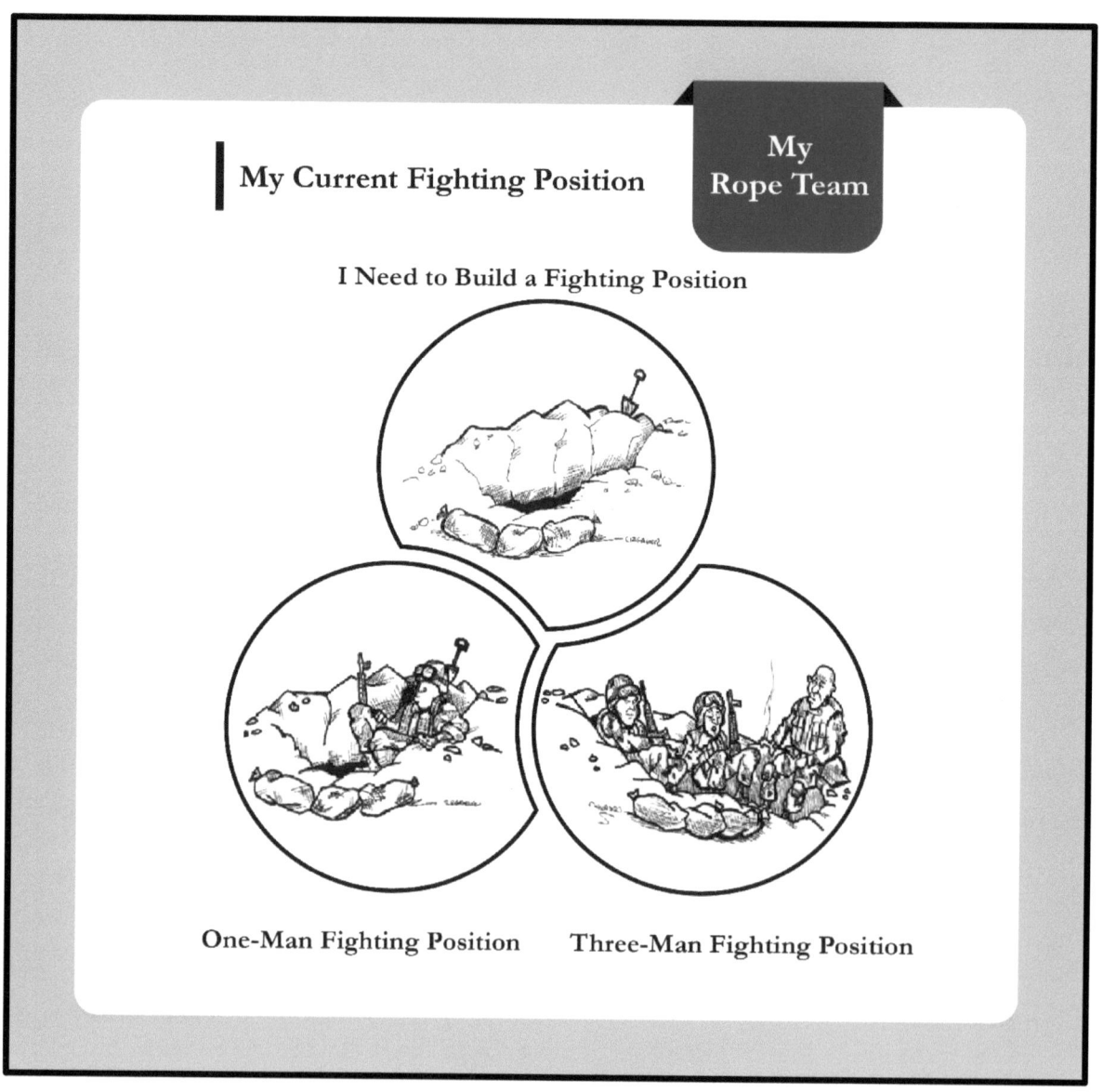

The Art of Medicine – A Warriors Profession™

Exercise 2. B: Depending on how you answered the question regarding your current fighting position in EXERCISE 2. A. You will **DEFINE** which of the following two (2) questions you must answer in Worksheet 2. B: Describing My Current Fighting Position. This learning process will help you better understand your current situation.

1) For those individuals who find themselves predominantly in a One-MAN FIGHTING POSITION, this is another exercise in self-reflection. We want you to **THINK** about why you find yourself fighting alone, using Worksheet 2. B (a): Describing My Current Fighting Position; first, **WRITE** why you find yourself in a One-MAN FIGHTING POSITION. Second, **WRITE** out the pros and cons of your situation. Is this your predominant fighting position, or just your current circumstances?

2) For those who have found their foxhole buddies, skip to Worksheet 2. B (b): Describing My Current Fighting Position, we want you to think of an occasion when you find yourself fighting alone. **DESCRIBE** why you fought alone and how you found your way out of the One-Man death trap. By reflecting on the situation, you can provide insight into fellow foxhole buddies and **ROPE TEAM** members.

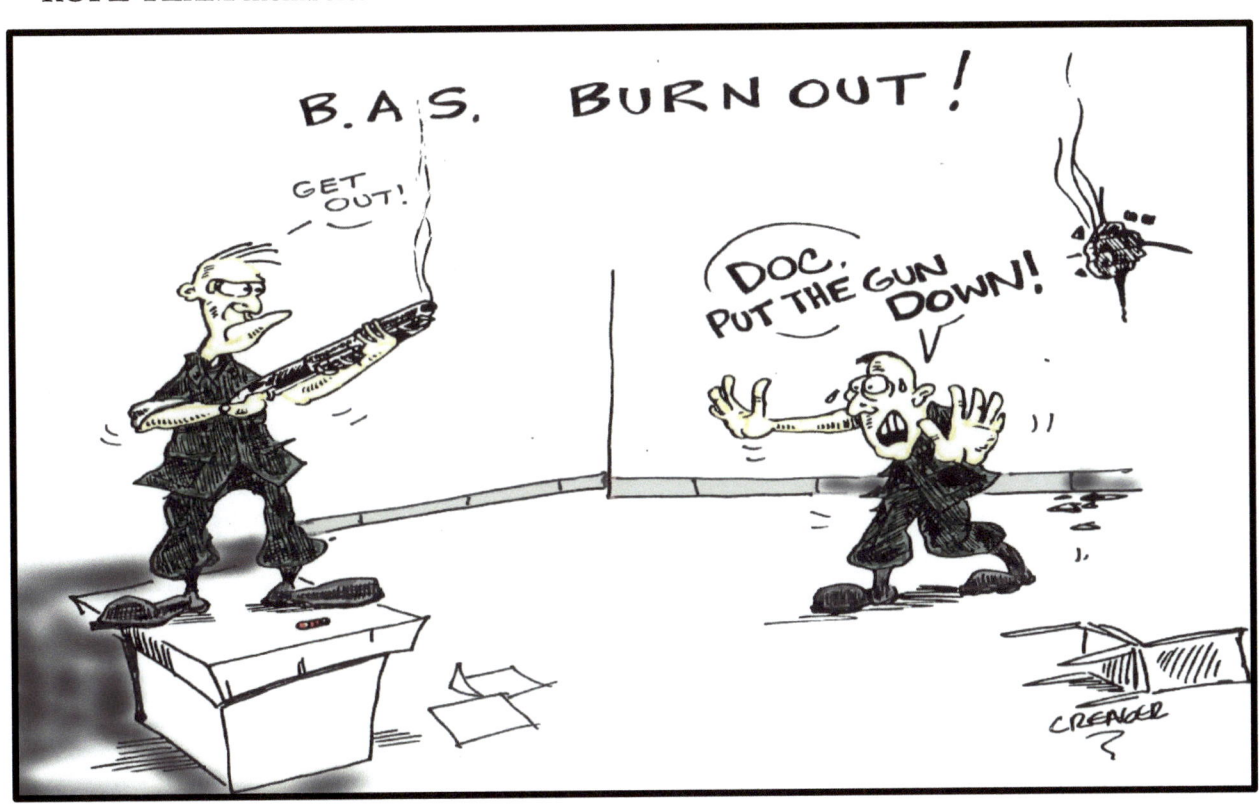

WORKSHEET 2.B: DESCRIBING MY CURRENT FIGHTING POSITION

My Current Fighting Position — My Rope Team

Reasons why you find yourself predominantly in a One-Man Fighting Positions?

Pro's and Con's of your particular Situation?

Copyright © 2024 Johnnie L. Gilpen Jr
Created by: Huma Rafeeq

Worksheet 2. B: Describing My Current Fighting Position

My Current Fighting Position

My Rope Team

Why did I find myself fighting alone, and how did I find my way out?

Copyright © 2024 Johnnie L. Gilpen Jr
Created by: Huma Rafeeq

Exercise 2. C: As you go forward before you attempt to build either a personal or professional **Rope Team**, you need to build your own mental Three-MAN FOXHOLE. This is an exercise in reflection and forethought. Our question to you is, WHOM do you want in your foxhole? WHOM do you TRUST to watch your back? These people do not have to have the same backgrounds or viewpoints as you. They do not have to be family, nor is knowing someone all your life or being a coworker a specific qualifying factor.

Inclusion criteria should include someone who knows your history and your goals. Someone who will encourage you! Someone who will hold you accountable when you are slacking – when you are being lazy! Choose those who will find motivation in your struggle when you are pushing yourself. Think about it – WHOM do you want to go to war with? In Worksheet 2. C: Identifying My Foxhole Buddies, **WRITE** your name in the top center circle and the names of your two (2) foxhole buddies in the other two (2) circles. ***Remember, the foxhole principle is reciprocal – meaning it goes both ways.*** (Goggins, 2022; Maxwell, 2004). Choose people you are willing to be the same kind of friend you are asking them to be.

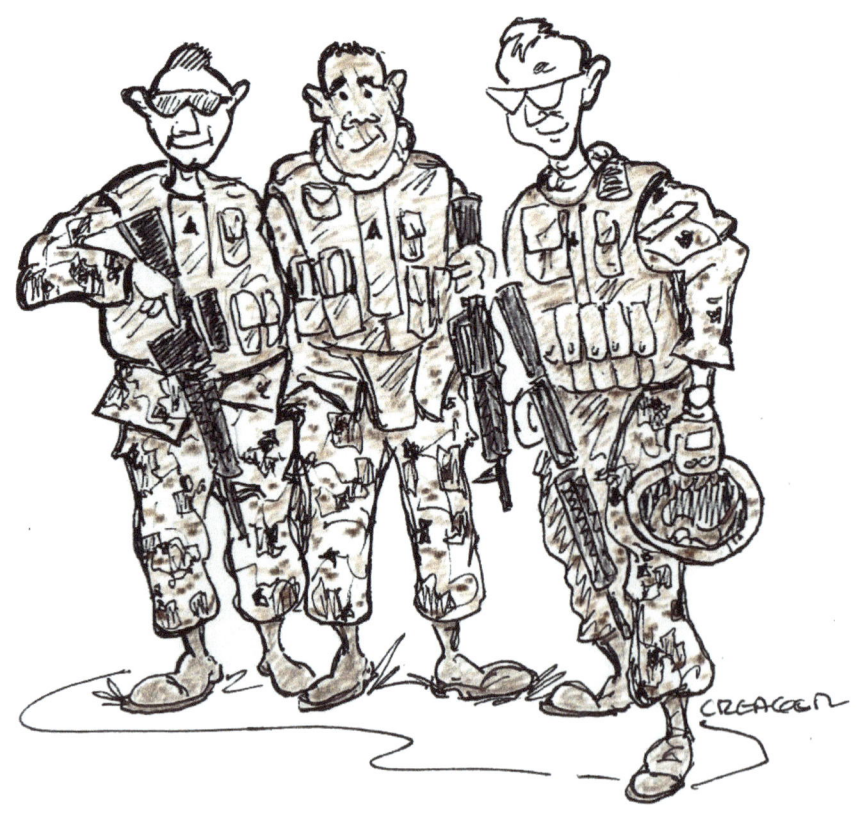

WORKSHEET 2. C: IDENTIFYING MY FOXHOLE BUDDIES

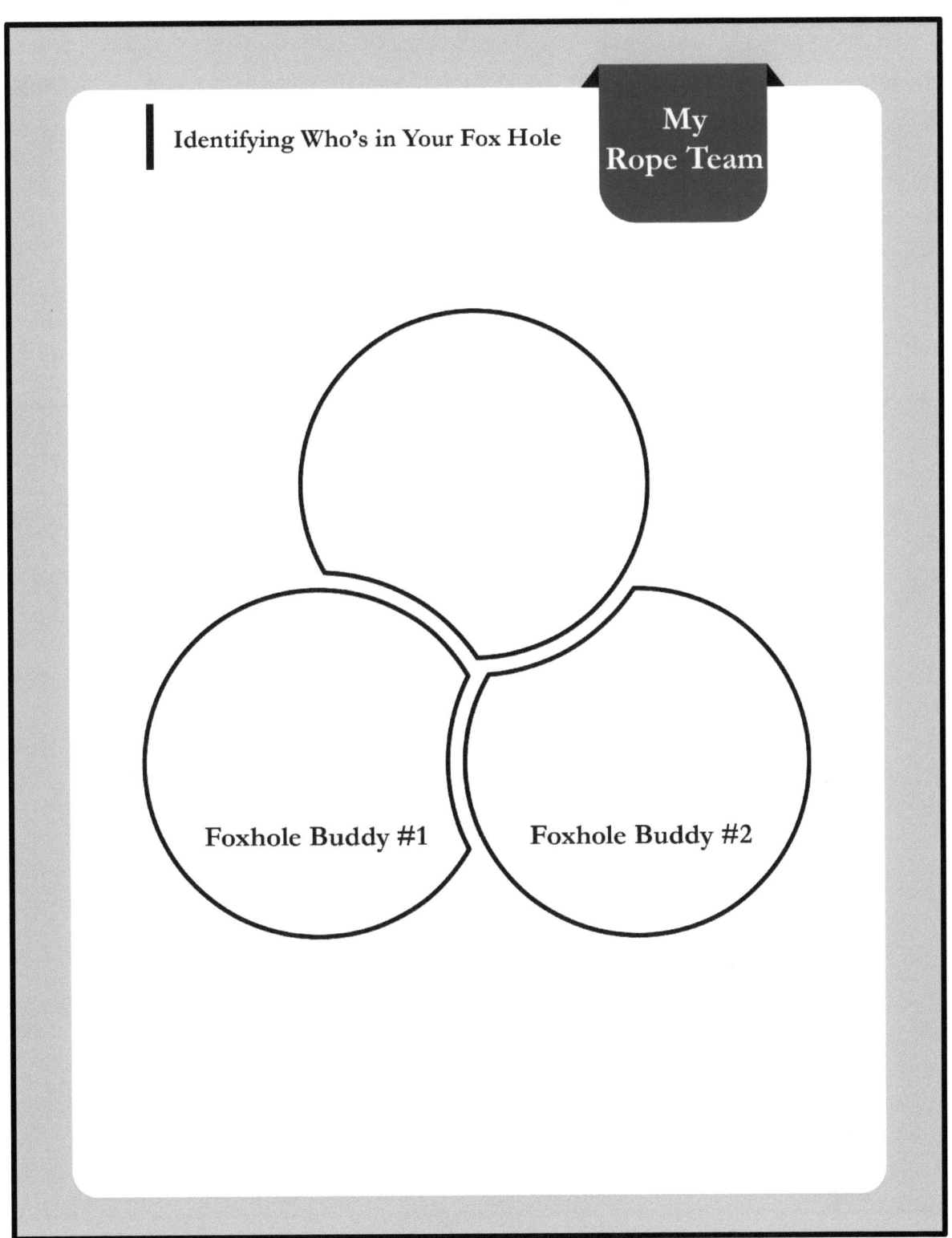

Exercise 2. D: In EXERCISE 2. C, you were asked to use the Foxhole Principle, discussed this in training, to **IDENTIFY** two (2) individuals you want in your mental foxhole to help you fight your battles with, who you want to go to war with. These buddies will help you fight your battles. Sometimes, the biggest fight… will be with yourself. They should be individuals willing to push you beyond the threshold of what you believe is possible. In this exercise, use Worksheet 2. D: Characteristics of My Foxhole Buddy # 1 & 2. **WRITE** their name in the top left-hand corner. **WRITE** WHY you chose these two individuals. Be detailed – **DESCRIBE** the characteristics you believe will help you accomplish your goals.

WORKSHEET 2. D: CHARACTERISTICS OF MY FOXHOLE BUDDY # 1

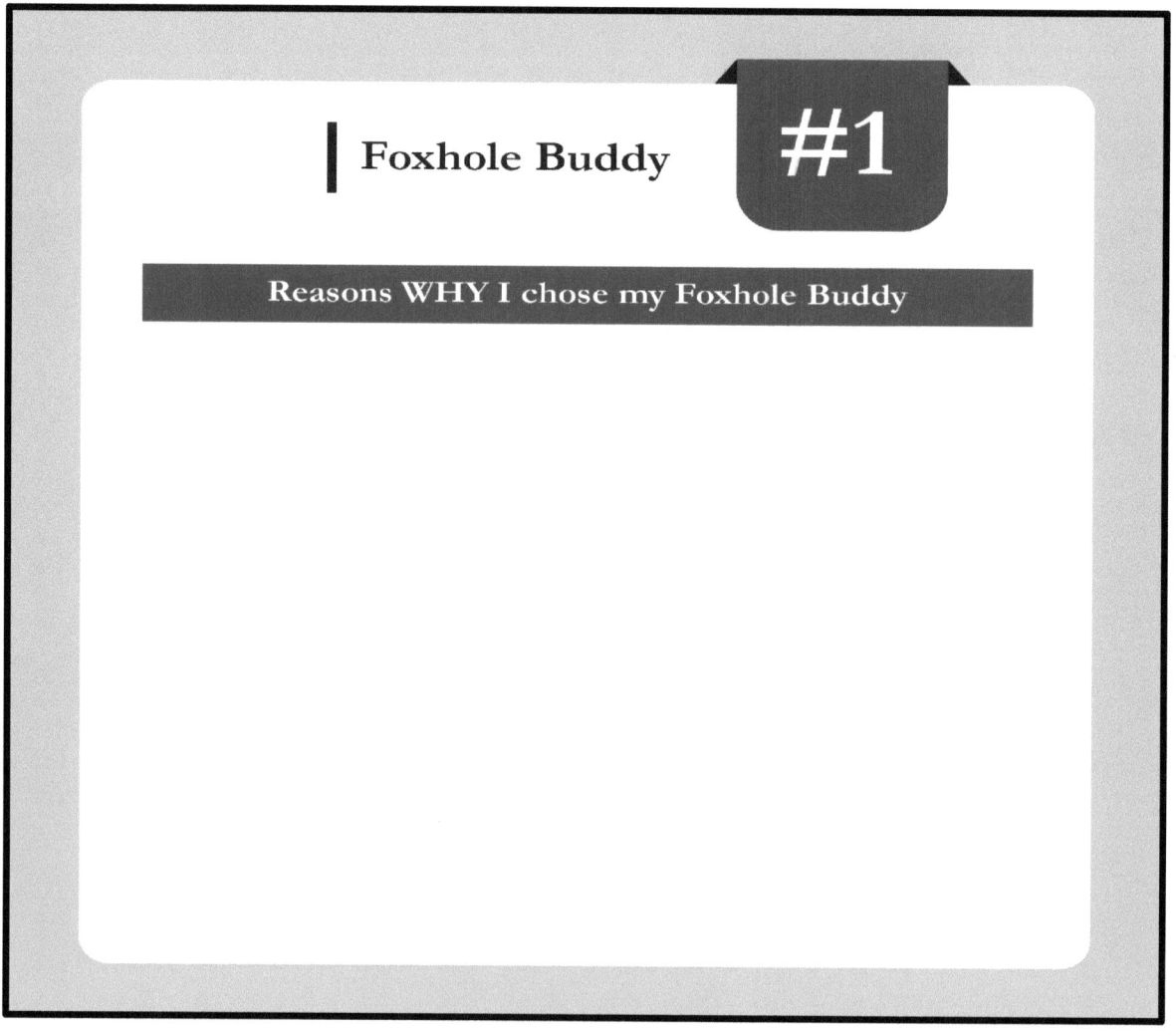

WORKSHEET 2. D: CHARACTERISTICS OF MY FOXHOLE BUDDY # 2

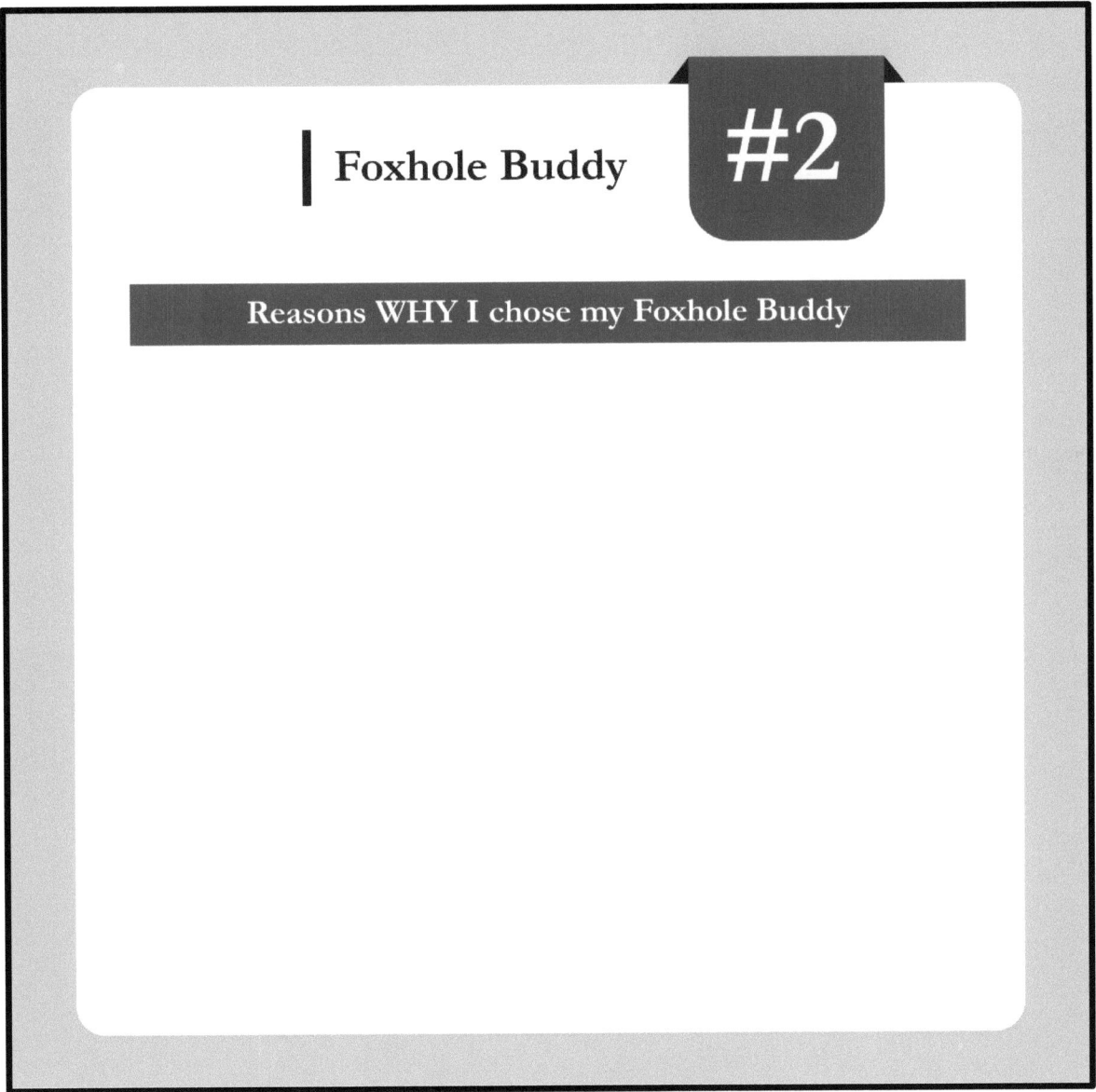

Exercise 2. E: You have received two (2) postcards – one (1) for each of your two (2) Foxhole Buddies in your Cookie Jar. Please **WRITE** a short postcard to each of them asking them to join you in your foxhole of life, using the information you wrote in EXERCISE 2. D, **TELL** them WHY you chose them and that you are willing to reciprocate the same. If you know their address, there is a box in front of the class where you can drop your postcard off, and we will mail it for you, or you can mail the card

yourself. By doing this, you declare your friendship and loyalty in writing. It is a positive affirmation to both you and your friends!

Exercise 2. F: If you use social media, please **IDENTIFY** the two (2) people in your foxhole. Use the following hashtags:

#FoxholeBuddyARTMED   #ARTMEDWarriorProf
#NoBarriersARTMED   #PTF-ARTMED.

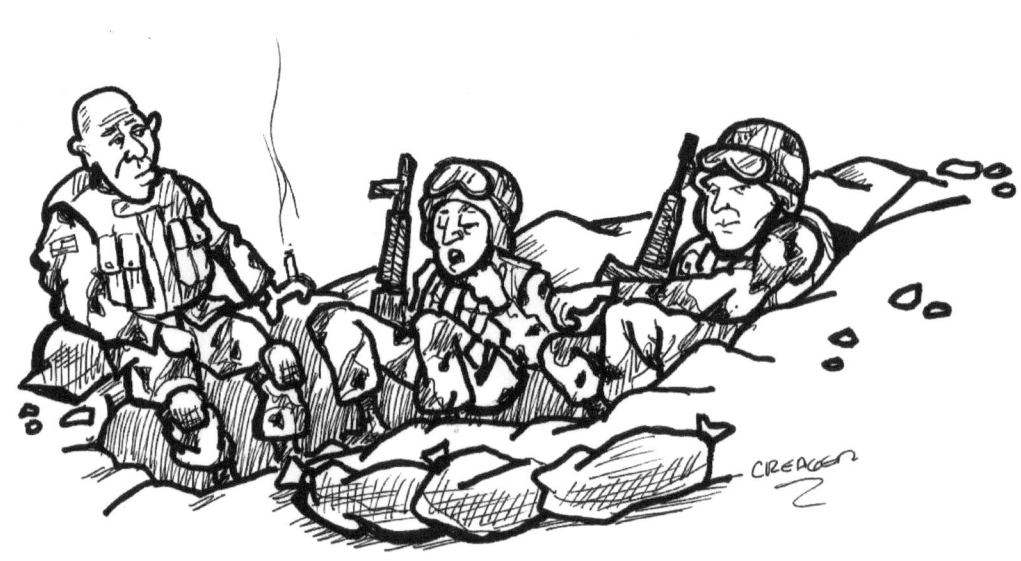

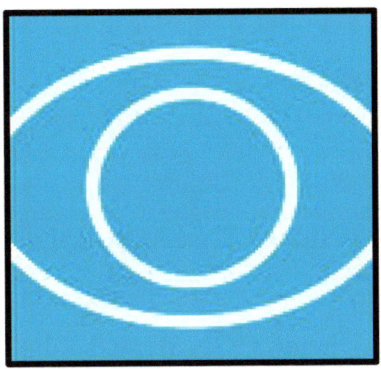

VISION

> "Values are your heart's deepest desires for how you want to behave as a human being. Values are not about what you want to get or achieve; they are about how you want to behave or act on an ongoing basis."
> — Russ Harris

Evolution Three: Defining Your Vision

The life element, **VISION**, aims to guide you in identifying your values and passions.

- What are the values that you live by?
- How did you develop these values?

Your **VISION** should serve as your life's compass and guide your decision-making process. Knowing your values and passion will help you react positively to the world around you.

For this evolution - **VISION**, you need to think about a goal or goals you have in life. To achieve this goal(s), you need a baseline from where to start, a foundation that helps distinguish who you are and how you perceive yourself – a statement that identifies your values and passions. The exercises in this evolution will help you determine the values you identify with, personally and professionally, and provide you with some tools to help serve as guides for the future. Developing this groundwork guides

HOW, WHERE, WHO, and WHEN to invest your time and energy. Once you have established your values and passion, share them with your rope team, foxhole buddy, family, coworkers, etc. ("Vision - No Barriers Warriors," 2020).

Evolution Three Objectives:

1. **IDENTIFY** the participant's core values by self-reflection on personal resiliency data points, summits, achievements, and obstacles. **CONSIDER** OBSTACLES the participant has overcome, is currently facing, and has yet to conquer.

2. The participants will **CREATE** their own *VISION CAIRN* using the data identified in OBJECTIVE 3.1.

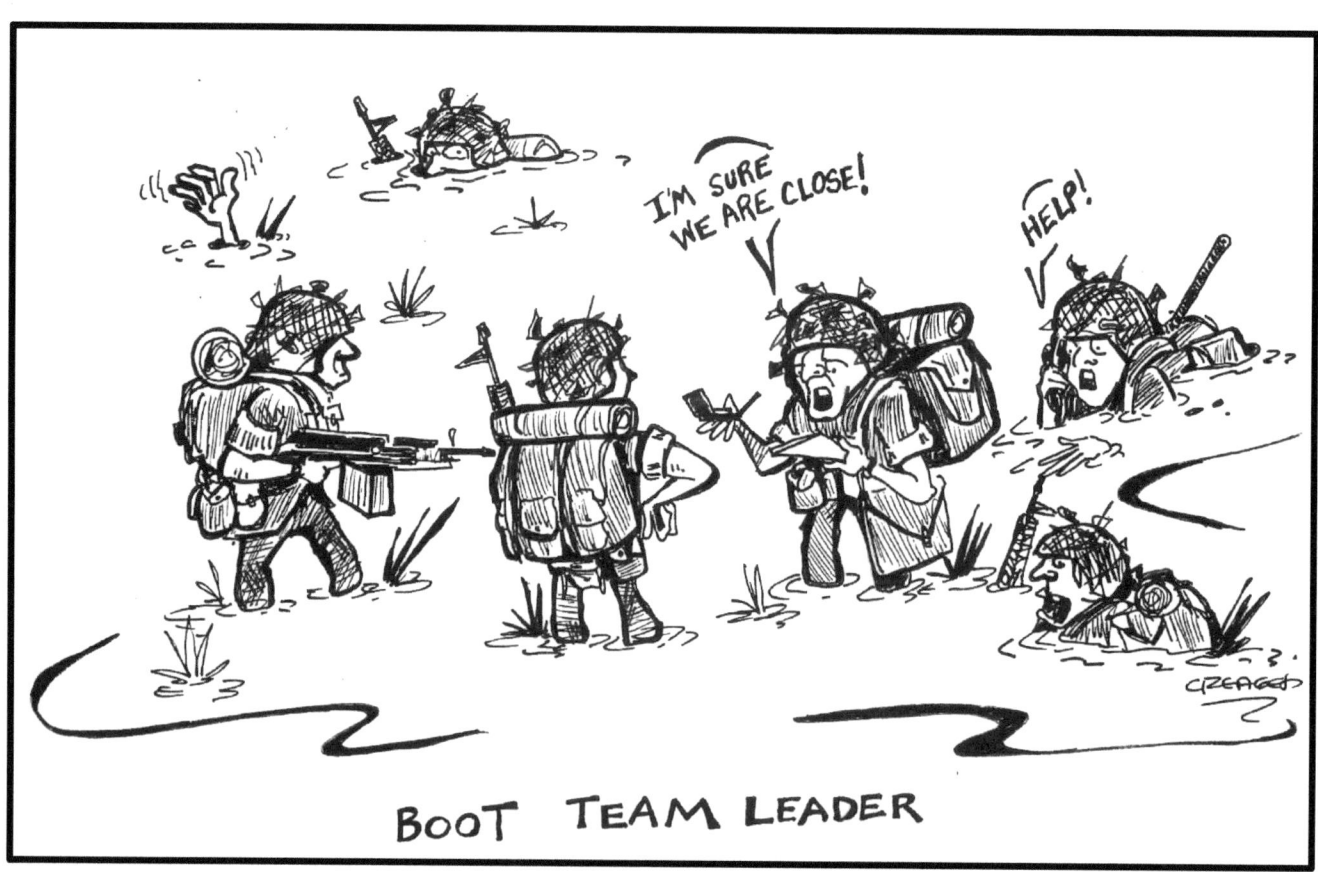

VISION

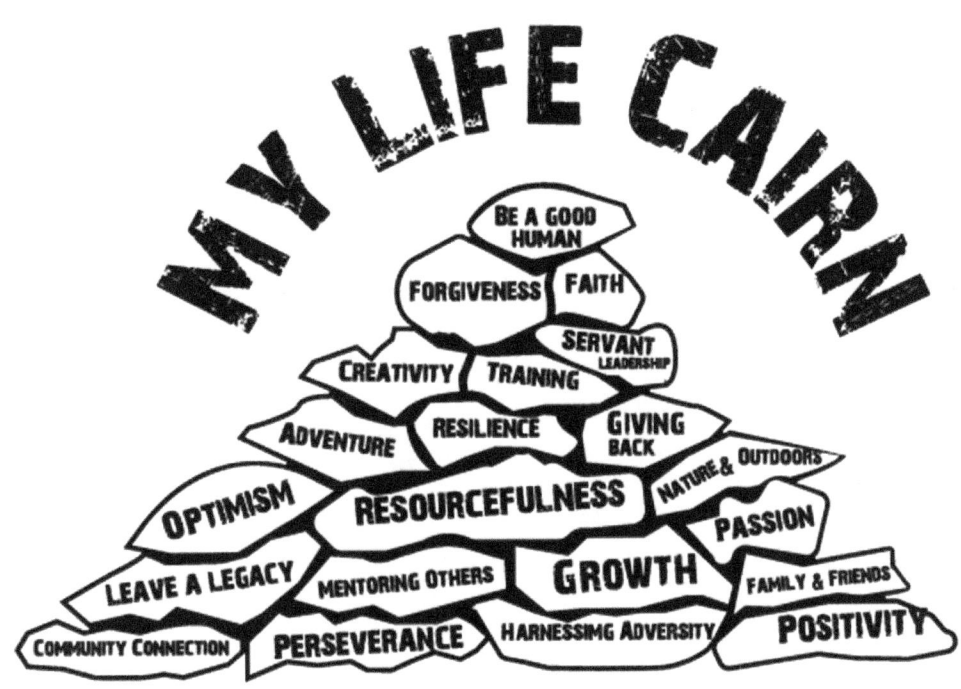

Evolution Three: Defining Your Vision

Evolution Three Exercises:

Exercise 3. A: In the military, taking a knee – refers to physically taking a knee while quickly setting security. The objective is to pause, take a breather, drink some water, pull out your map, mentally step back, and consider the tactical environment… hopefully to gain some perspective on your operational situation. In this exercise, we are asking you to mentally take a knee. Pull out your mental map of life – checking the route you have plotted for the journey and the road to your ultimate destination in life.

Make a quick gut check. Again, we ask you to be honest: Does the road you are currently traveling on align with your values? Do you even know what your values are? Have you ever sat down and physically written your values down on paper?

In the **VISION** Chapter of *What's Within You*, the authors Tom Lillig and David Shurna (Lilling & Shurna, 2020c) pose the following questions to help readers discern if the reader's vision aligns with their individual values:

1. What inspires you and gets you up in the morning?
2. What are the things that bring you joy?
3. What activities, experiences, and people help you feel grounded and connected in your life?
4. What do you need to let go of (values, beliefs, behaviors) to integrate your answers to the questions above into your daily routines?
5. How big of a change are you willing to make to integrate your answers to the questions above into your daily routines?

Keeping these questions in mind, **WRITE** 20-25 values you identify in the space provided in the My Values Mind Mapping Box worksheet. If you have difficulty finding words to **DESCRIBE** your specific values, we have provided a prompt box for Exercise 3. A: Prompt Box with examples. As you go through the exercise, keep the questions above in mind.

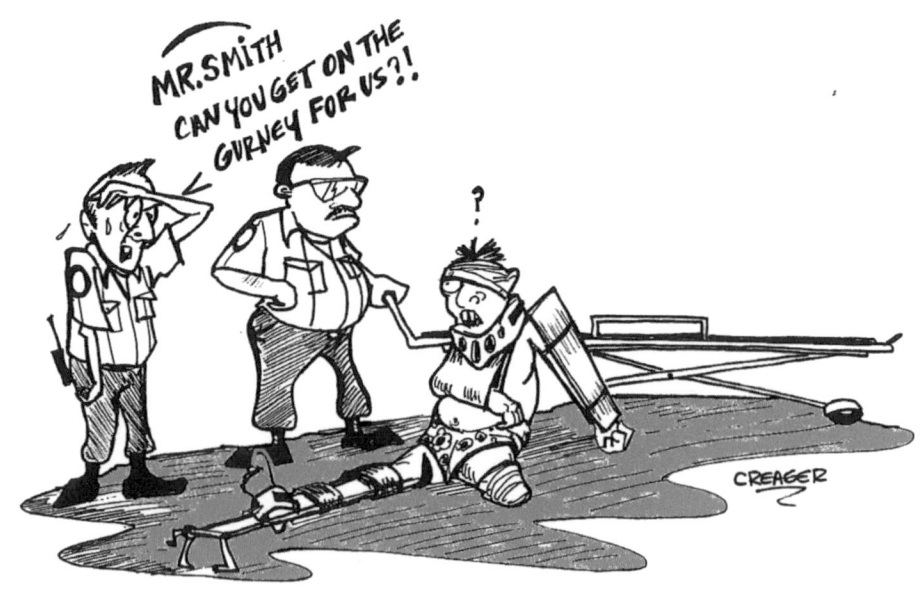

Exercise 3. A Prompt Box

My Vision

- Achievement
- Community
- Connection
- Courage
- Dependability
- Education

- Faith
- Friendship
- Giving
- Growth
- Health & Fitness
- Humor
- Independence

- Justice
- Kindness
- Leadership
- Love
- Mentoring
- Peace
- Resilience
- Resourcefulness
- Security
- Sincerity
- Spontaneity
- Understanding
- Training
- Wealth

- Adventure
- Compassion
- Creativity
- Enthusiasm

- Family

- Good Health

- Honesty
- Integrity

- Learning

- Mentorship
- Perseverance
- Resiliency

- Servant Leadership

- Success
- Uplifting Others
- Trust
- Wisdom

- Art
- Confidence
- Curiosity
- Excellence

- Forgiveness

- Gratitude

- Humility
- Intelligence

- Leave a Legacy

- Optimism
- Positivity
- Respect

Resilience

WORKSHEET 3, A: MY VALUES BRAIN MAPPING BOX

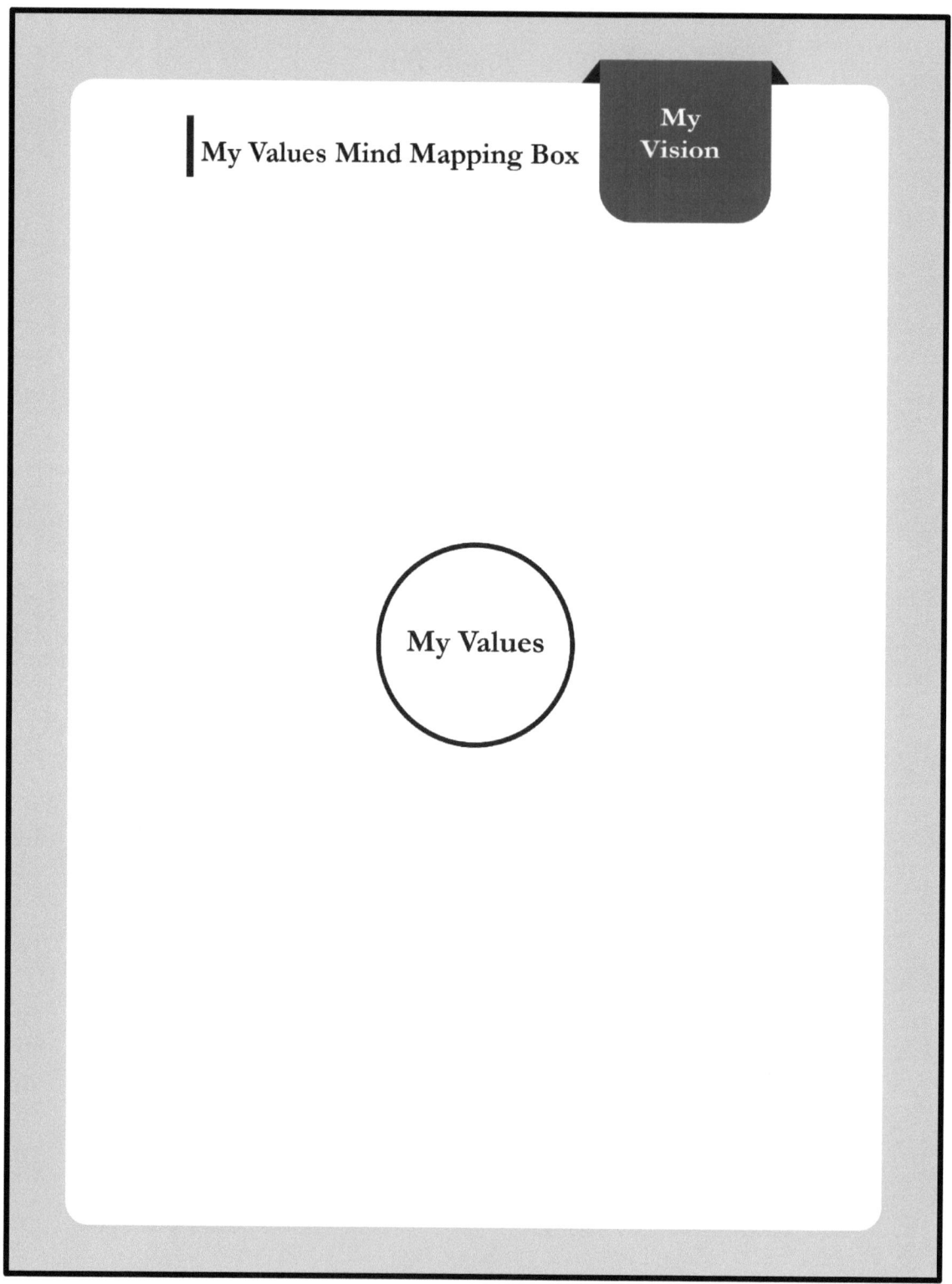

Exercise 3. B: Part of taking a knee is looking at your map – your map of life – and evaluating whether you are on the correct heading. When hiking and unsure exactly where you are, you can always return to your last known point on the trail. Often, the trail is marked with cairns, particularly when it is difficult to follow due to extreme terrain.

CAIRNs are man-made piles or stacks of rocks used to mark the trail, a turn in the trail, or often the top of a mountain. Often, you can only navigate the trail from cairn to cairn. The same concept can be used for life by creating mental cairns. Like physical rocks on the trail, our values guide our life's actions – specifically, our life goals.

In EXERCISE 3. B, with the values you **IDENTIFIED** in Worksheet 3. A: My Values Mind Mapping BOX, place them in the empty rocks in the VISION CAIRN on Worksheet 3. B: Building My Vision Cairn, building your mental cairn. The cairn can be used as a fallback when you get lost, are confused, or need to reset. Remember to structure it like building a physical cairn – the most significant values are used as the base to support the rest of your values. (Refer to the example below)

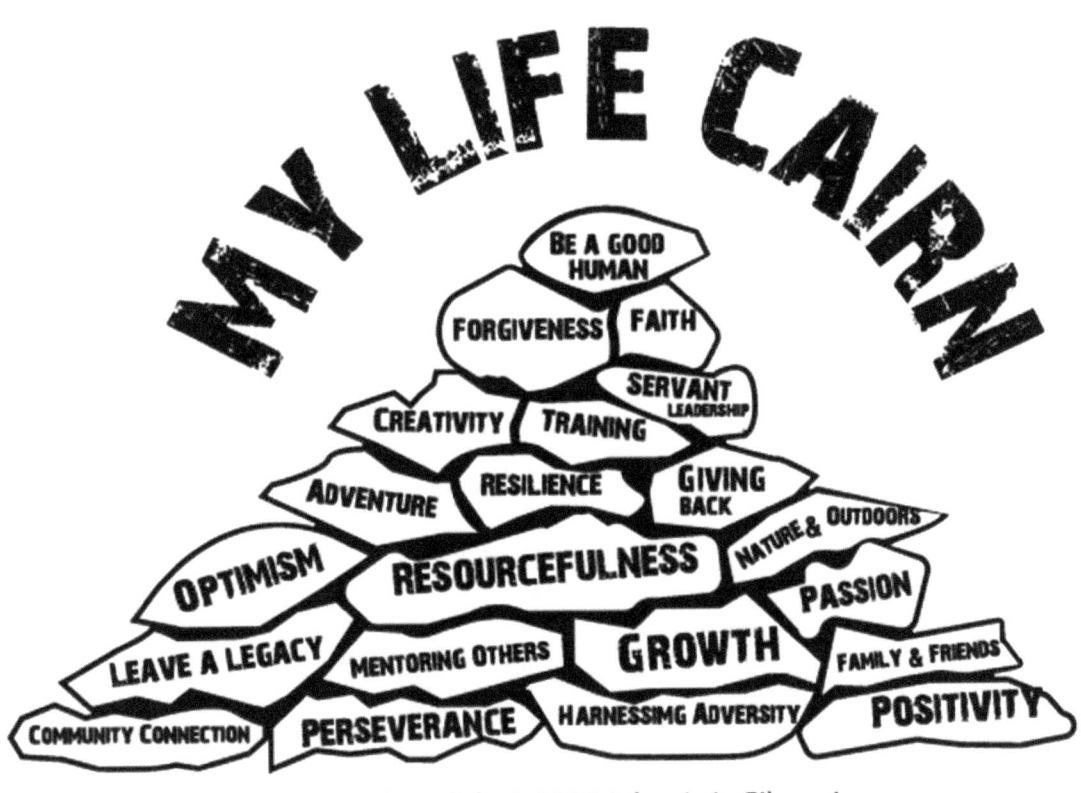

Copyright © 2024 Johnnie L. Gilpen Jr
Created by: Huma Rafeeq

WORKSHEET 3. B: BUILDING MY VISION CAIRN

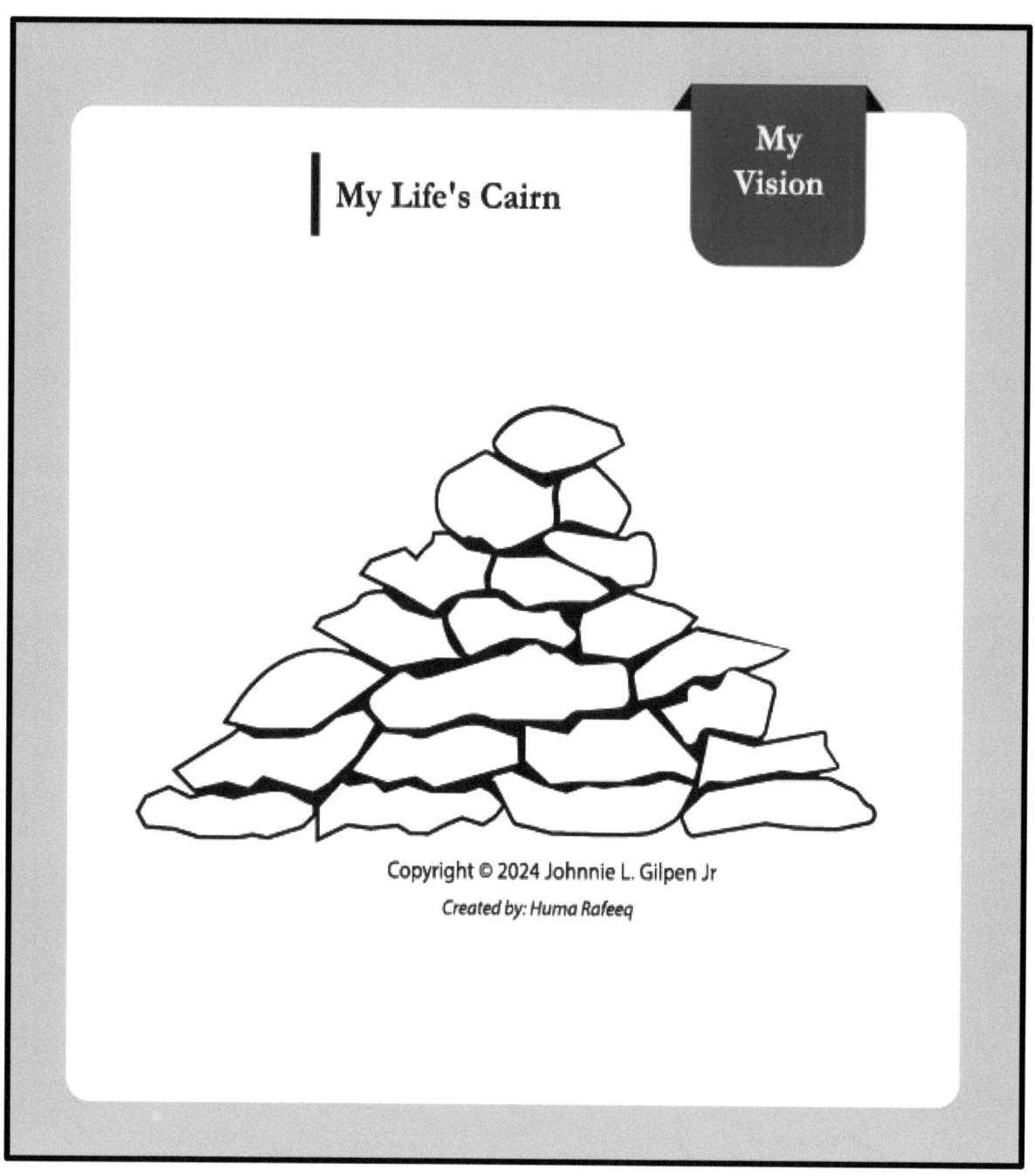

Alternative Option – **DRAW** your own personal VISION CAIRN in the space provided below.

Exercise 3. C: In your Cookie Jar is a blank MY VISION CAIRN postcard. **TRANSCRIBE** the values you placed in Worksheet 3. B: Building My Vision Cairn. You can pull out this MAP when you take a mental knee. It is a reference to help you find your way back to your center when you feel you have lost your way.

Developing a Warrior's Mindset to Cultivate Resilience and Professional Longevity

Exercise 3. D: Now that you have created your own VISION CAIRN, you can use it to help guide you and provide a point to fall back on when you need to regroup. Let us put the cairn into a framework for our future. To do that, we want you to **CONSIDER** the three (3) following questions and **PROVIDE** three answers using your VISION CAIRN to help guide you.

1. I want to continue to learn and grow in the following three areas –
   1.1

   1.2

   1.3.

2. Which builds upon my passions for –
   2.1

   2.2

   2.3

3. By continuing to learn and grow in these areas, I will have a greater impact on the things I care about the most:
   3.1

   3.2

   3.3

The Art of Medicine – A Warriors Profession™

Now, using this information and your VISION CAIRN, fill in the following statement:

My values of … _____, _____, and _____, are the foundations of this ongoing development.

By integrating these things into my everyday activities, I will be remembered as someone who:

My values of _____, and _____, are the foundation of this ongoing growth and resilience transformation.

REFERENCES

De Sena, J., & Pence, L. (2021). *10 Rules For Resilience*. Harper Collins.

Goggins, D. (2022). Evolution No.6. In *Never Finished*. Lioncrest Publishing.

Maxwell, J. C. (2004). The Foxhole Principle. In *Winning With People* (pp. 133-143). Thomas Nelson.

Paine, A. B. (2018). *Mark Twain, a Biography, Vol. 3 of 4: The Personal and Literary Life of Samuel Langhorne Clemens (Classic Reprint)*. Forgotten Books.

Rope Team - No Barriers Warriors. Barriers (Ed.), *No Barriers*. Ft Collins: No Barriers.

Summits - No Barriers Warriors. (2020). In Barriers (Ed.), *No Barriers*. Ft Collins: No Barriers.

Publisher Contact Information

For information regarding publishing, please reach out to one of the following

Email: info@8404publishing.com

Mailing address: 8404 Publishing LLC
    7997 Alfadale Street
    Union City, Oklahoma 73090

    www.8404publishing.com

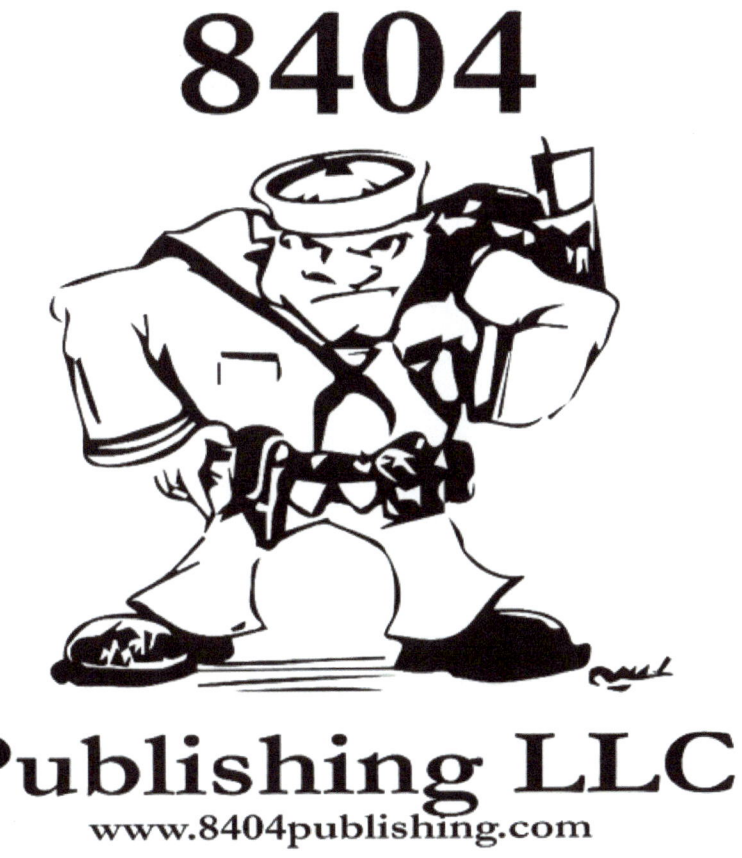

Developing a Warrior's Mindset to Cultivate Resilience and Professional Longevity

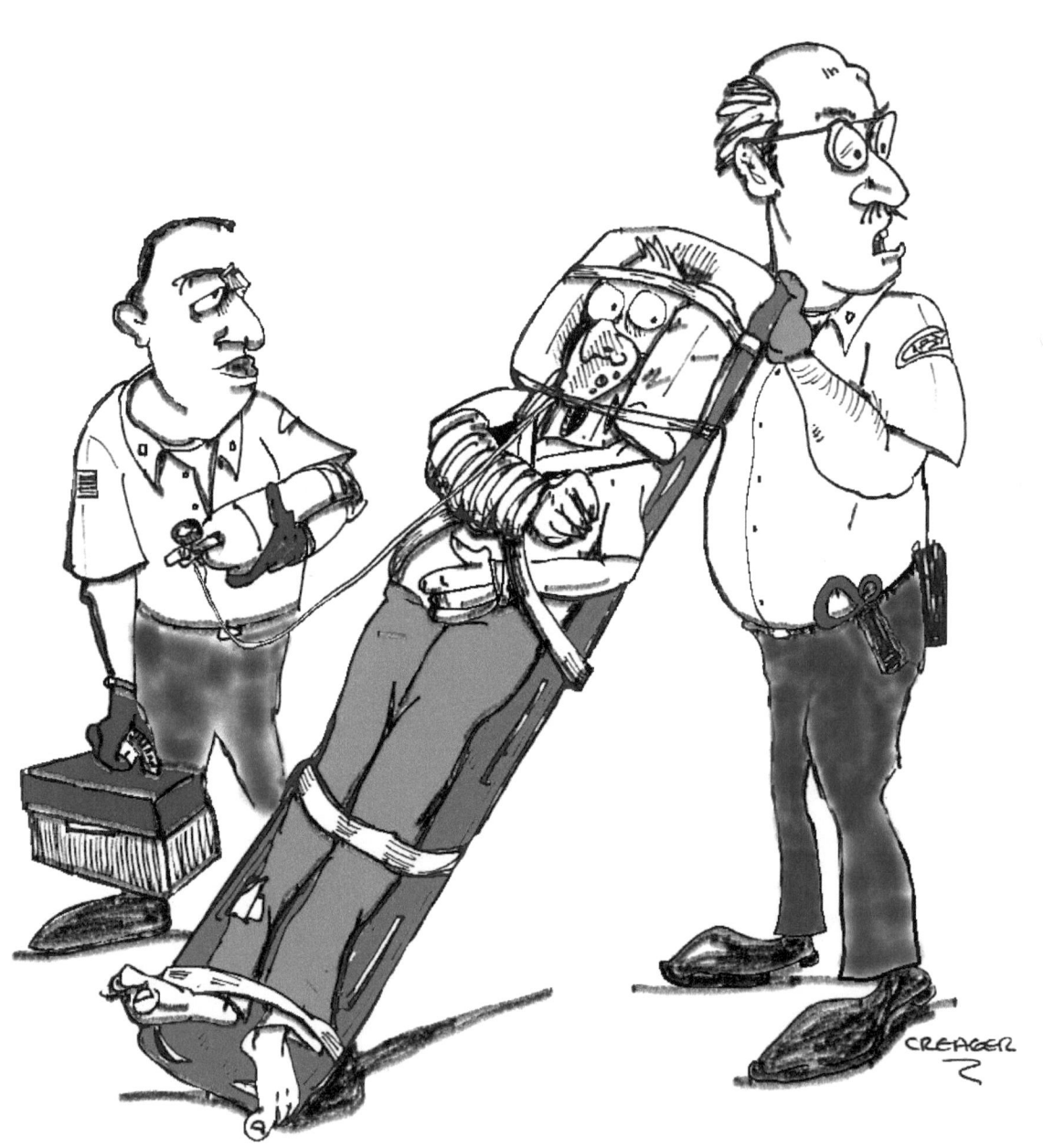

Perseverance

APPENDIX

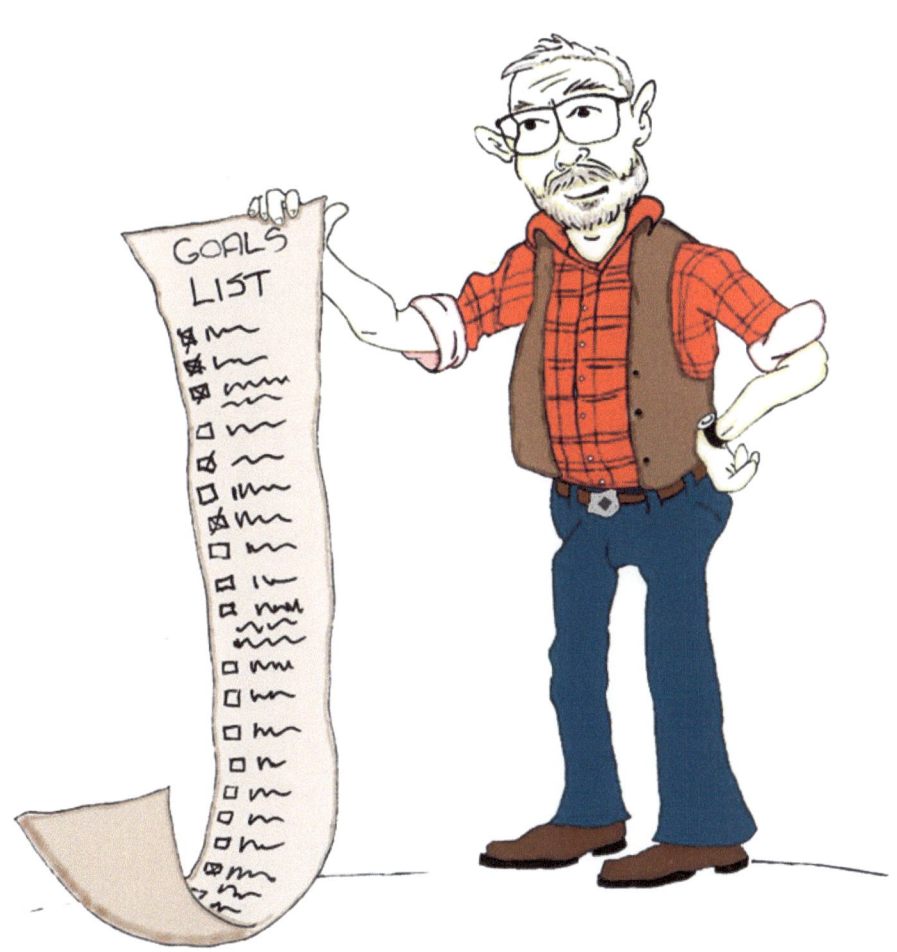

Appendix A: Book List

Campbell, J. (1990). *The Hero's Journey.* New World Library.

Easter, M. (2021). *The Comfort Crisis.* Rodale Books.

Epstein, D. (2019). *Range: Why Generalists Triumph in A Specialized World.* Penguin Random House.

Evans, J. B. (2016). *Mountain Vision: Lessons Beyond the Summit.* Touchwood Press.

Evans, J. B. (2020). *Climbing Through Storms: Managing Adversity in a VUCA World.* Mountain Vision Publishing.

Ferris, T. (2017). *Tribe of Mentors: Short Life Advice from the Best in the World.* Houghton Mifflin Harcourt Publishing.

Frankl, V. E. (1959). *Man's Search for Meaning.* Beacon Press

Frisella, A. (2020). *75 Hard: A Tactical Guide to Winning the War with Yourself.*

Googins, D. (2018). *Can't Hurt Me: Master Your Mind and Defy the Odds.* Lioncrest Publishing.

Goggins, D. (2022). *Never Finished.* Lioncrest Publishing.

Hill, N. (1937). *Think and Grow Rich.* Penguin Random House INC.

Lillig, T. & Shurna, D. (2020). *What's Within You – Your Roadmap to Living Life with No Barriers.* Kenilworthlore Publishing.

Maxwell, J. C. (2004). *Winning With People.* Harper Collins Leadership.

Pressfield, S. (2002). *The War of Art: Break Through the Blocks and Win Your Inner Creative Battles.* Black Irish Entertainment LLC.

Stoltz, P. G. (1997). *Adversity Quotient: Turning Obstacles into Opportunities.* John Wiley & Sons, INC.

Warren, R. (2012). *The Purpose Driven Life: What on Earth A, I Here For.* Zondervan.

Weaver, T. (2019). *The Evolution of a Leader.* Kindle Direct Publishing

Weaver, T. (2020). *All My Best: Wisdom and Encouragement for A Better Life.* Terry Weaver Books.

Weihenmayer, E. (2002). *Touch The Top of The World.* Penguin Group.

Willink, J. (2020). *Discipline Equals Freedom Field Manual MK1-MOD1.* St. Martin's Press.

Appendix B: OK First Responder Wellness Division

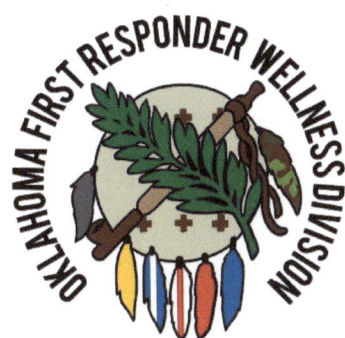

The Oklahoma First Responder Wellness Division was unanimously passed and written into the Oklahoma State Statute in 2022. We are the only Full-Time state-funded PEER program committed to supporting our first responders' physical, mental, and spiritual well-being. Here's a brief overview of the services we offer:

- Stress Management Massage Chairs: Specially designed for anxiety relief.
- Sleep Treatment Beds: Aimed at addressing sleep-related issues from trauma exposure.
- Hyperbaric Chamber: Providing therapeutic benefits for mental well-being and cognitive health.
- Brain Mapping/Neuro Feedback: Utilizing advanced techniques to develop targeted therapeutic interventions & strategies to address trauma-related issues non-invasively.
- EMDR Therapy: Known for its effectiveness in treating trauma by helping First Responders process & overcome trauma.
- First Responder Financial Classes: Courses are built and led by professionals to help manage debt, investing, budgeting & retirement.
- Statewide physical fitness & nutritional program: There is something for everyone regardless of your condition, from Functional Fitness, Ruck/Walk groups, & Yoga for First Responders.
- Critical Incident Stress Management: We offer one-on-one and group peer support, defusing & debriefings after a traumatic incident(s).
- Mental Health Training: Specifically designed for First Responders & the battles faced throughout your career.
- Statewide Services: We are in OKC, but our Team is embedded across our State.

Our OKC office is staffed with certified peer members & trauma counselors, ensuring dedicated and trusted support. If you've experienced sleep deprivation or noticed a change in your behavior after a critical incident or a combination of incidents, our offerings are designed to help combat those symptoms.

We can bring all our mental & physical training to you and your agency. All services are FREE, and your privacy is protected under Oklahoma State statute 12:2506.2. It is entirely normal to be affected by our career choices and what comes with them, but it DOES NOT have to define you. Every OKFRWD Team member has been there, and together, we will help find a positive outcome for you and your FAMILY.

At your service,
The Oklahoma First Responder Wellness Division Team

For appointments, training requests, or to learn more, don't hesitate to get in touch with Hannah Henshaw at hannah.henshaw@dps.ok.gov or call (405)482-2731.

Appendix C: Worksheets

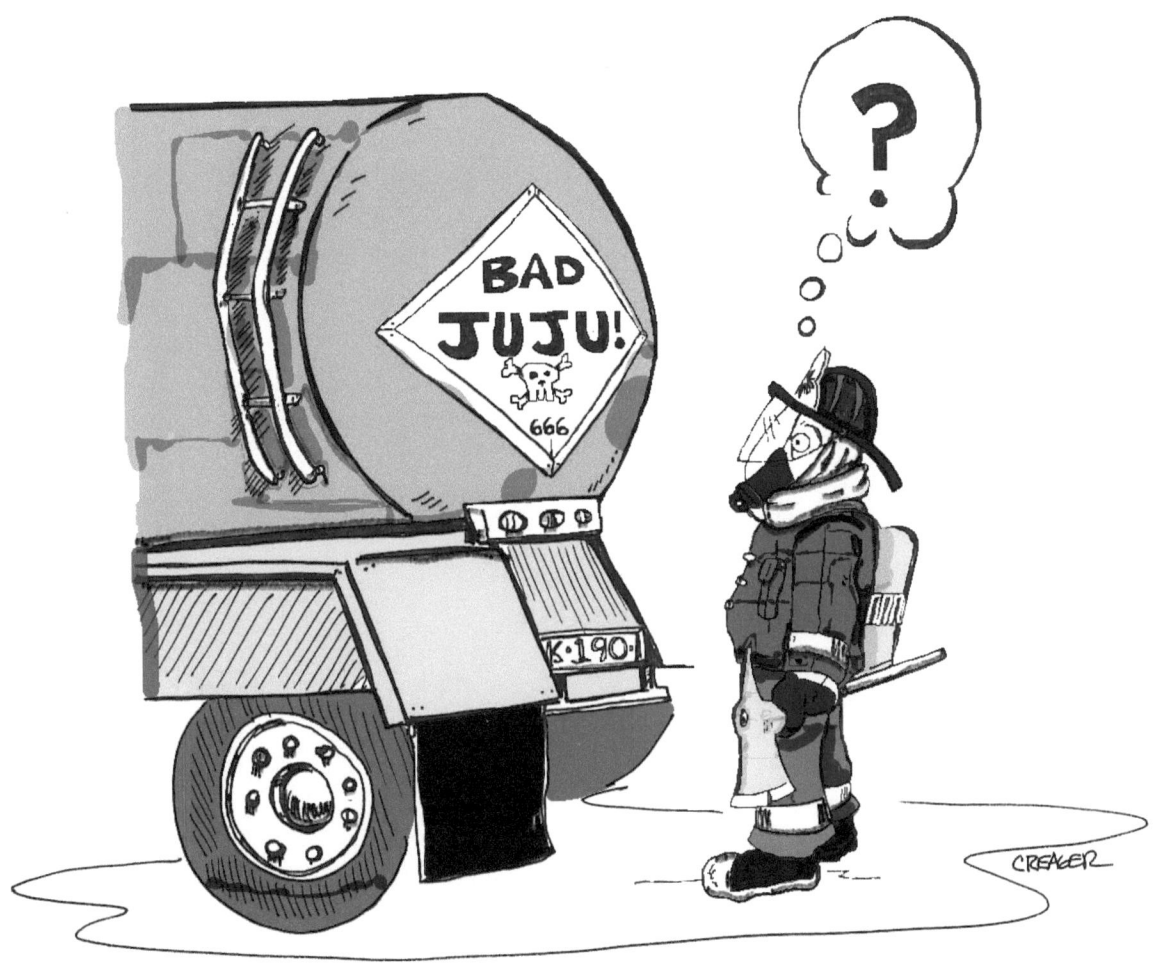

Worksheet 1. A: Identifying Your Life's Summits

My Summits

Identifying Your Life Summits

1.

2.

3.

4.

5.

6.

Perseverance

Worksheet 1. B: Resilience Data Point #1

Resilience Data Point #1

Your Summit #1

When?

Where Were You?

Who Were You With?

Why Was This Summit So Significant?

What Obstacles Did You Overcome?

Worksheet 1. B: Resilience Data Point #2

| Resilience Data Point #2 |

Your Summit #2

When?

Where Were You?

Who Were You With?

Why Was This Summit So Significant?

What Obstacles Did You Overcome?

Perseverance

Worksheet 1. B: Resilience Data Point #3

Resilience Data Point #3

Your Summit #3
When?
Where Were You?
Who Were You With?
Why Was This Summit So Significant?

What Obstacles Did You Overcome?

Worksheet 2. A: Identifying My Current Fighting Position

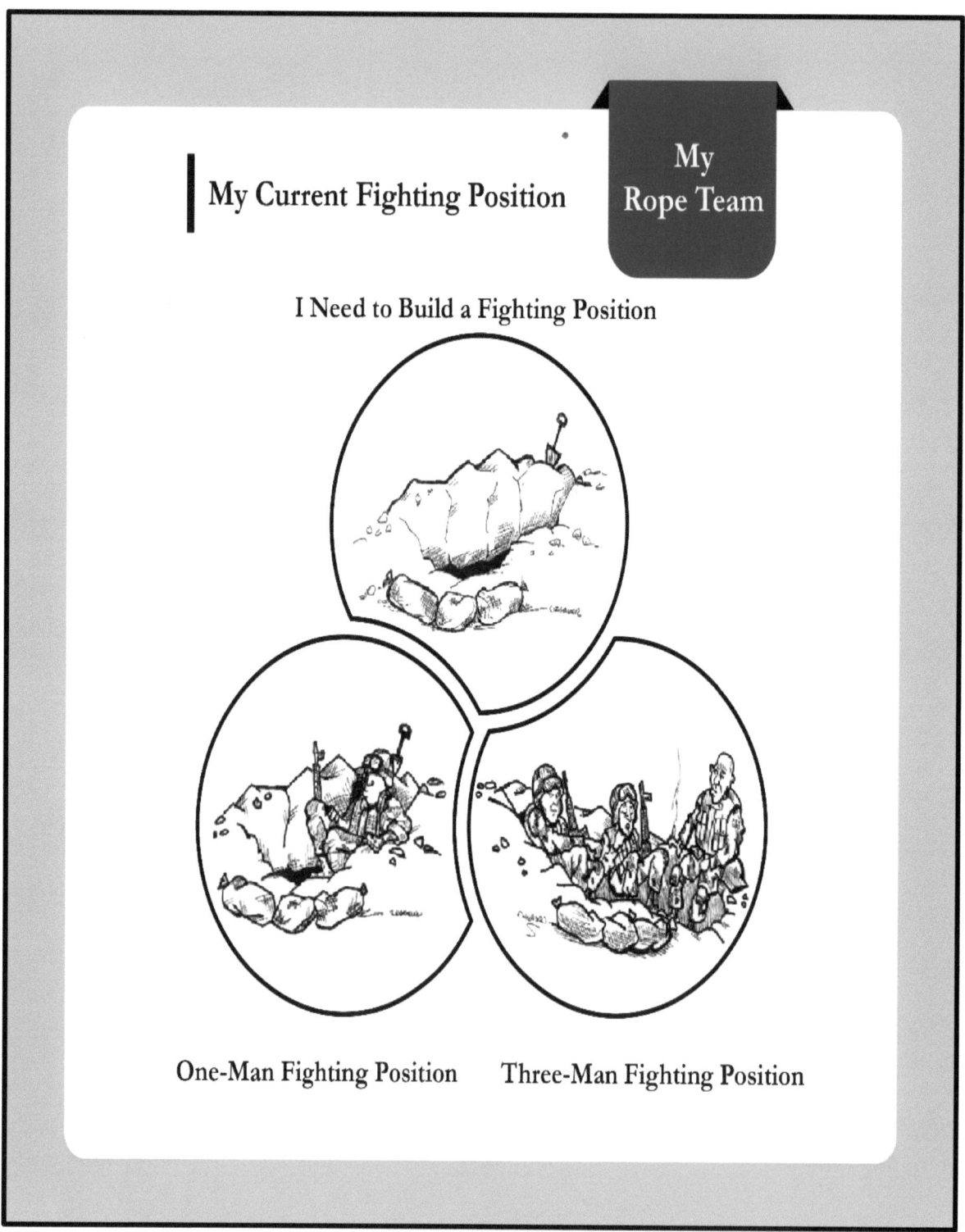

Worksheet 2. B: Describing My Current Fighting Position

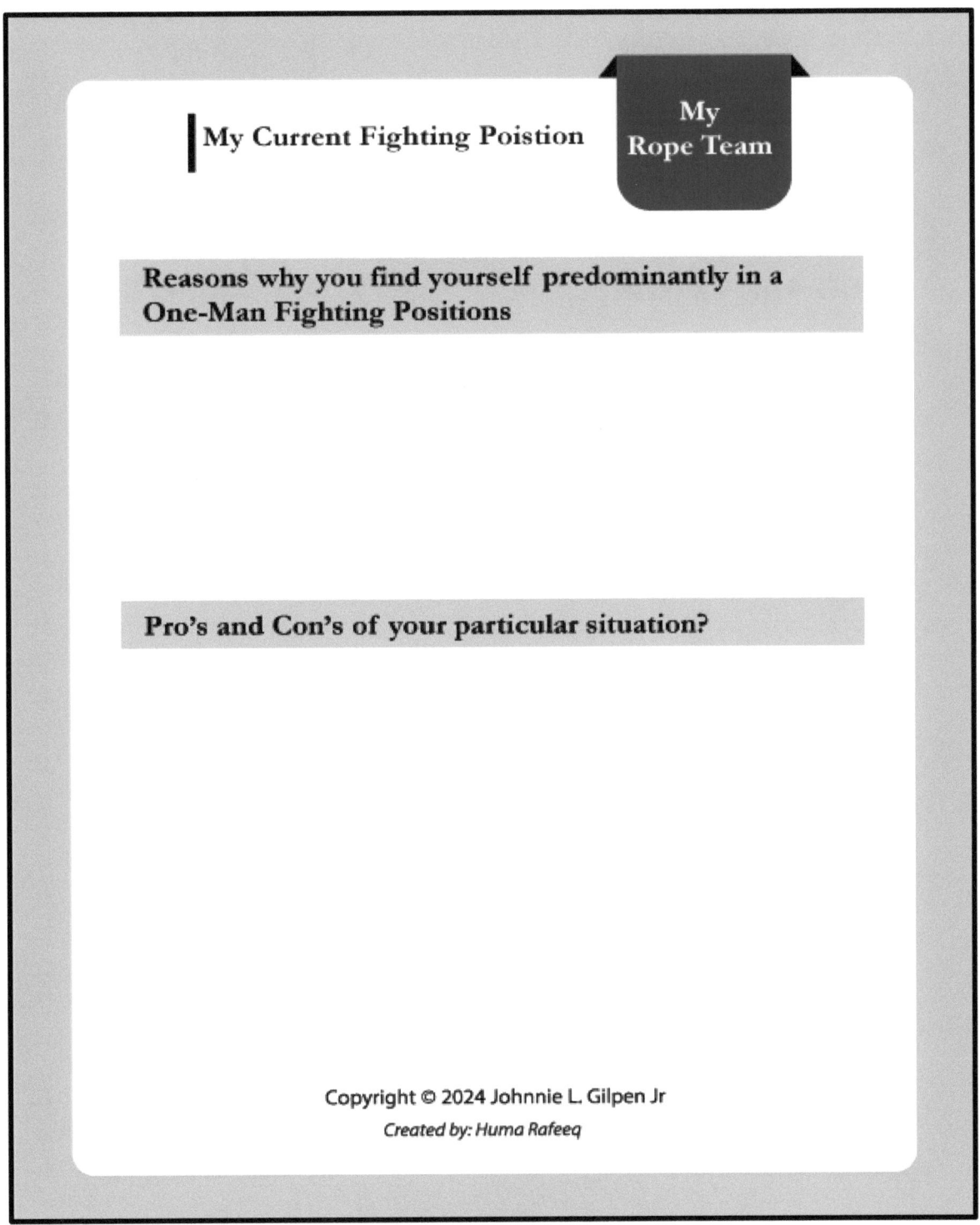

Worksheet 2. B: Describing My Current Fighting Position

My Current Fighting Position

My Rope Team

Why did I find myself fighting alone, and how did I find my way out?

Copyright © 2024 Johnnie L. Gilpen Jr
Created by: Huma Rafeeq

Worksheet 2. C: Identifying Who's In My Foxhole

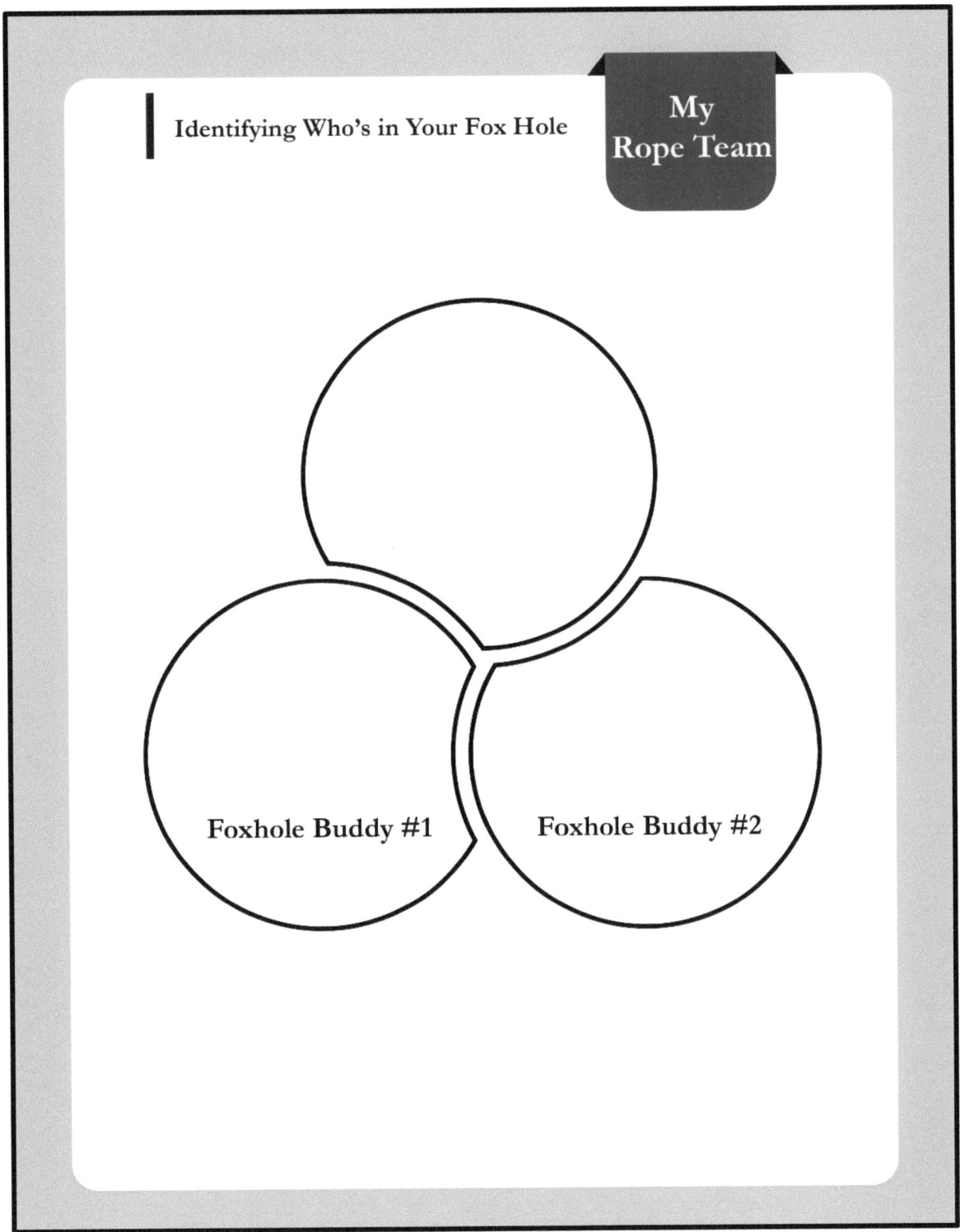

Worksheet 2. D: Characteristics of My Foxhole Buddy # 1

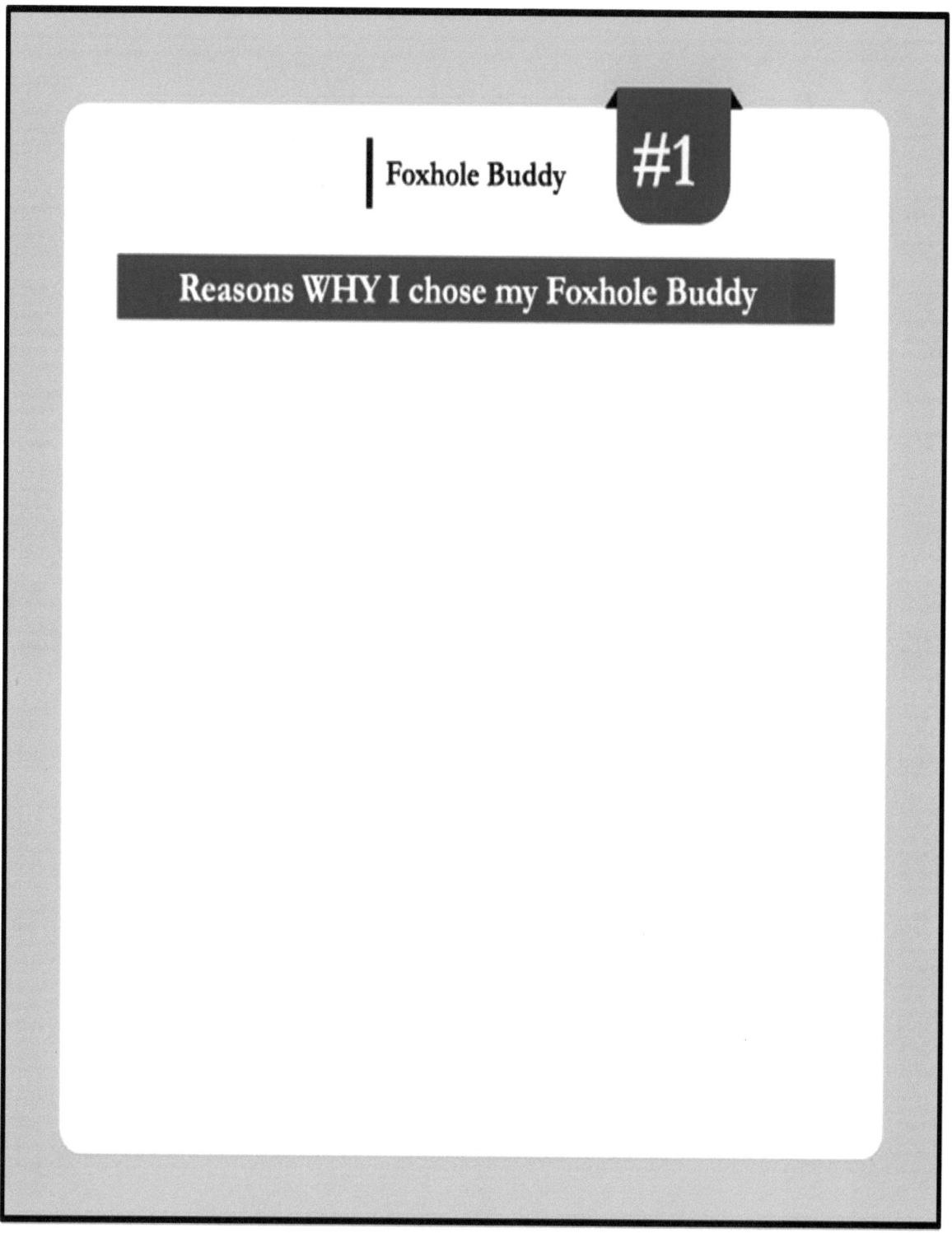

Worksheet 2. D: Characteristics of My Foxhole Buddy # 2

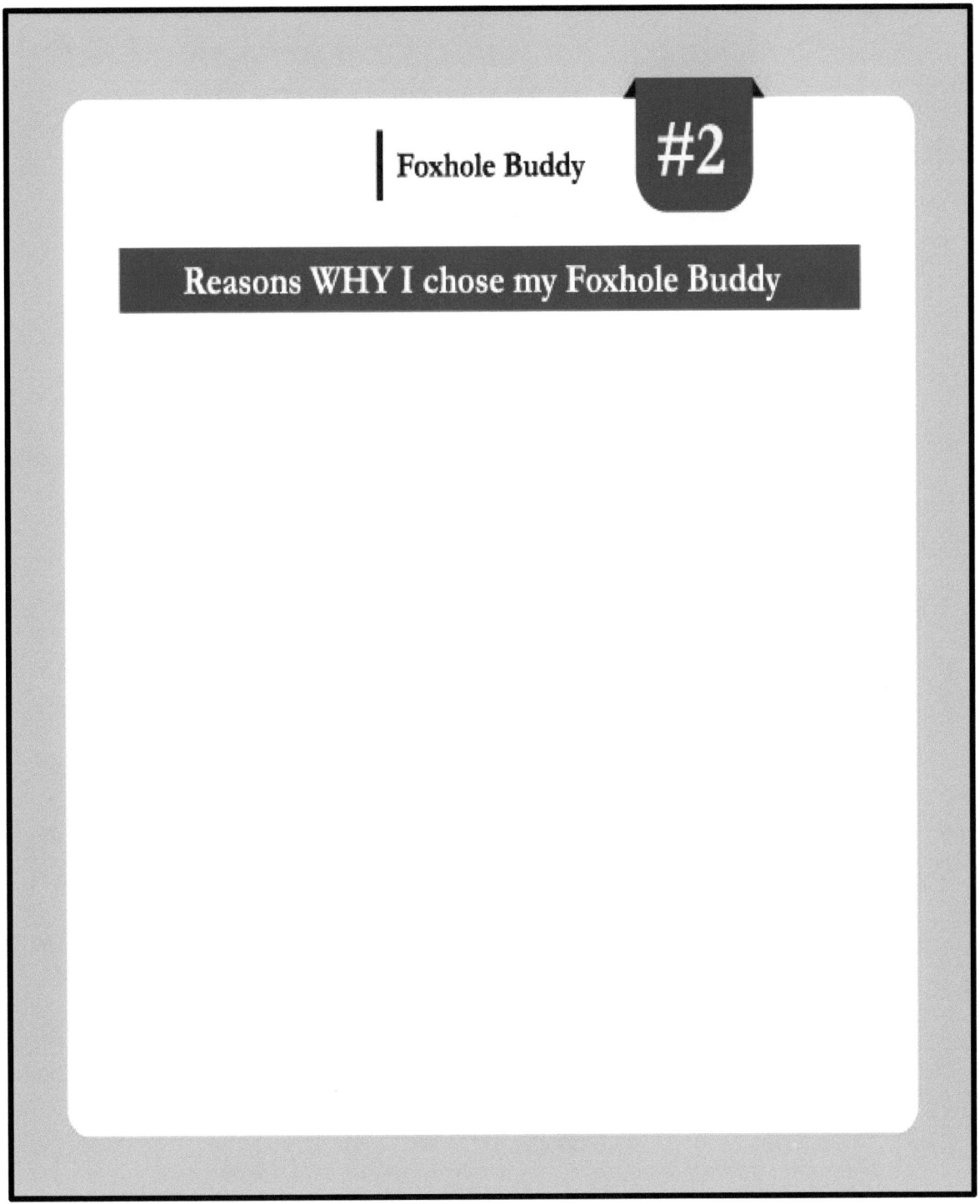

Exercise 3. A: Prompt Box

Exercise 1. A Prompt Box

My Vision

- Achievement
- Adventure
- Art

- Community
- Compassion
- Confidence
- Connection
- Courage
- Creativity
- Curiosity
- Dependability
- Education
- Enthusiasm
- Excellence

- Faith
- Family
- Forgiveness
- Friendship
- Giving
- Good Health
- Gratitude
- Growth
- Health & Fitness
- Honesty
- Humility
- Humor
- Independence
- Integrity
- Intelligence

- Justice
- Kindness
- Leadership
- Learning
- Leave a Legacy
- Love
- Mentoring
- Mentorship
- Optimism
- Peace
- Perseverance
- Positivity
- Resilience
- Resiliency
- Respect
- Resourcefulness
- Security
- Servant Leadership
- Sincerity
- Spontaneity
- Success
- Training
- Uplifting Others
- Understanding
- Trust
- Wealth
- Wisdom

Perseverance

Worksheet 3. A: My Values Brain Mapping Box

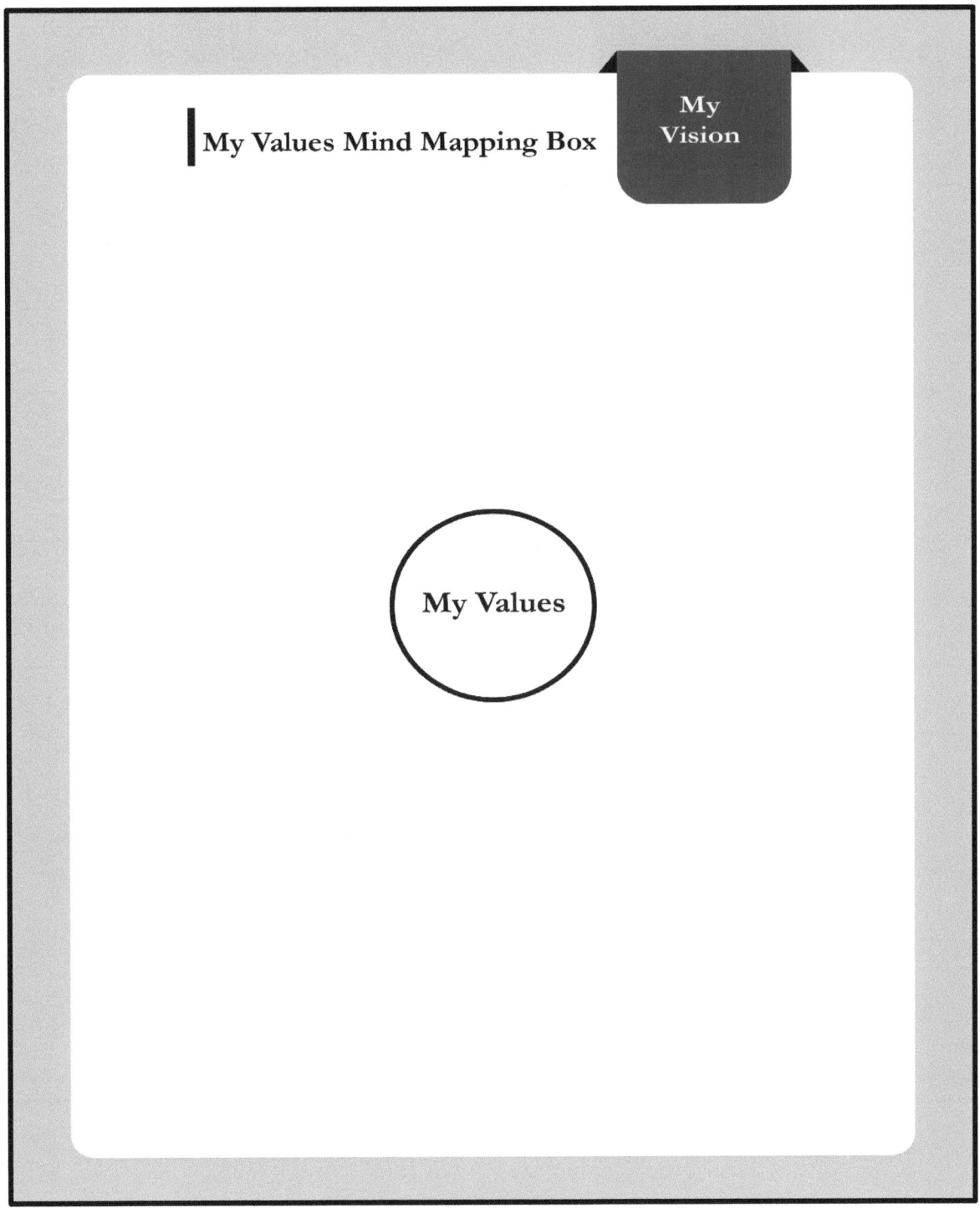

Worksheet 3. B: Building My Vision Cairn

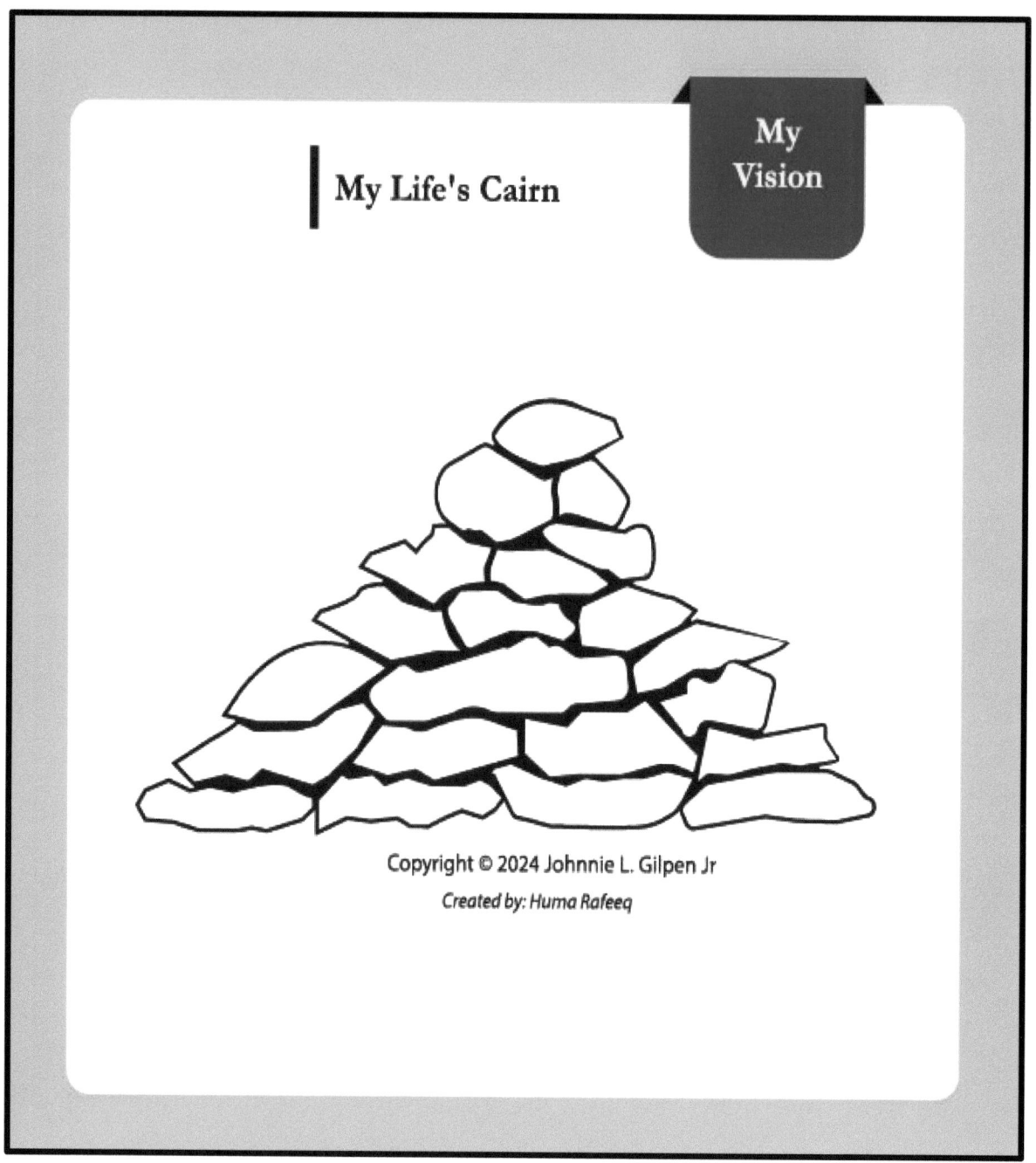

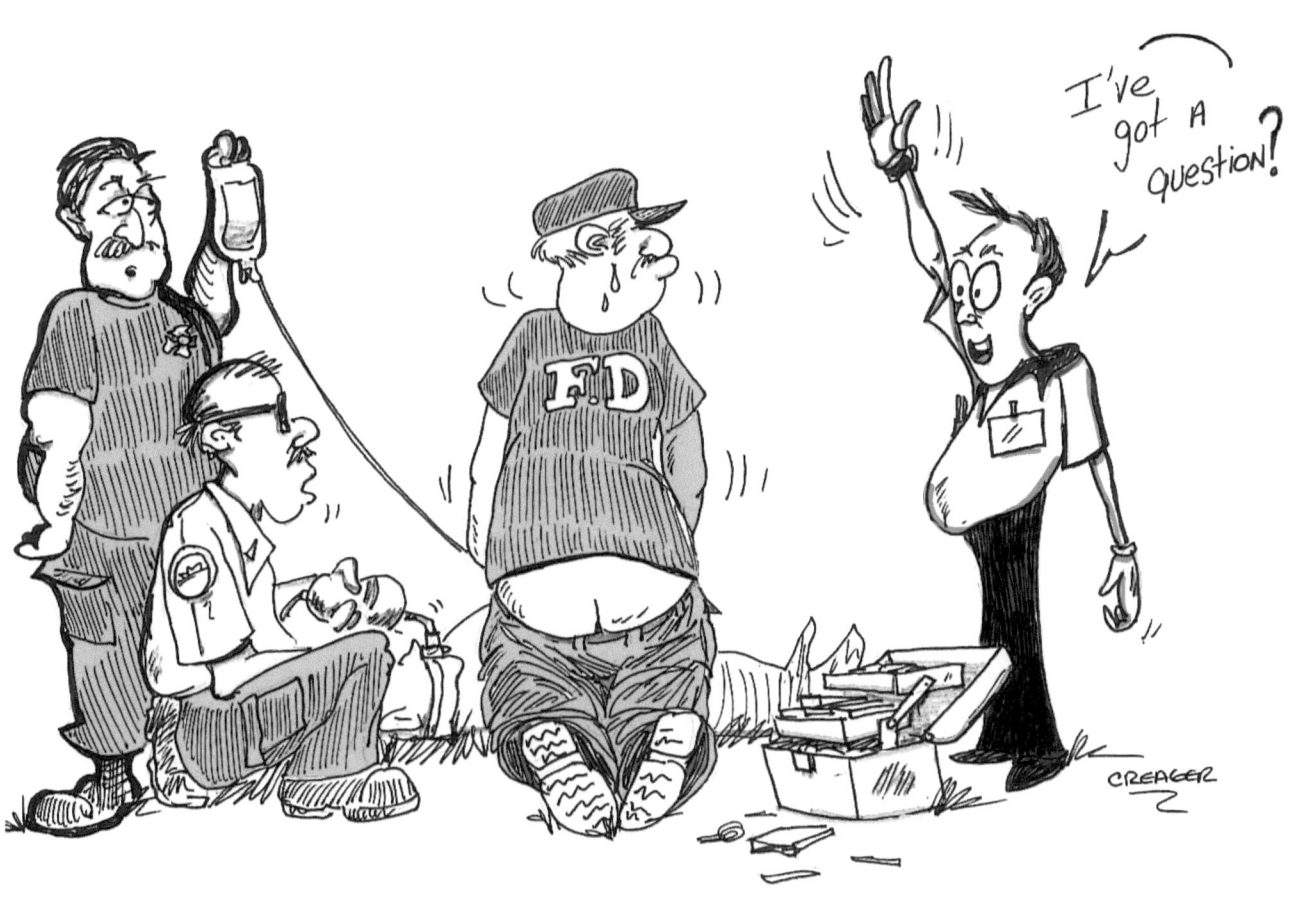

www.ingramcontent.com/pod-product-compliance
Lightning Source LLC
Chambersburg PA
CBHW041546220426
43665CB00002B/48